HEALTHQUEST
Total Wellness for Body, Mind & Spirit
STAYING STRONG

D0735225

HEALTH QUEST
Total Wellness for Body, Mind & Spirit

STAYING STRONG

Reclaiming the Wisdom of African-American Healing

EDITED BY SARA LOMAX REESE AND KIRK JOHNSON

WITH THERMAN EVANS, M.D.

AN AVON BOOK

The alternative healing methods described in this book are not intended as a substitute for medical advice from your physician. Always consult your doctor before beginning any new regimen that can impact your health. The publisher assumes no responsibility for any result derived from the implementation of the methods described herein.

AVON BOOKS, INC.
1350 Avenue of the Americas
New York, New York 10019

Copyright © 1999 by LEVAS, Inc.
Published by arrangement with LEVAS, Inc.
Library of Congress Catalog Card Number: 99-94878
ISBN: 0-380-79402-0
www.avonbooks.com/wholecare

First WholeCare Printing: September 1999

WHOLECARE TRADEMARK REG. U.S. PAT. OFF. AND IN OTHER COUNTRIES, MARCA REGISTRADA, HECHO EN U.S.A.

Printed in the U.S.A.

OPM   10   9   8   7   6   5   4   3   2

Contributors

Contributing Reporters and Writers
Kellye Davis
Glenn Ellis
Egypt Freeman
Gerda Gallop
K. Anoa Monsho
Darlene E. Paris
TaRessa Stovall

Contributing Editors
Valerie Boyd
Tamara Jeffries

Illustration
Kamela Eaton

Photography
William Richardson

Acknowledgments

When *HealthQuest* started in January 1993, many people asked the question: Why is there a need for a black health magazine? We know now what we knew then: we have inherited a rich and unique history that has left its imprint on our genes, our psyche and our spirit. By understanding this legacy we have the power to transform the future.

Six years later, and 500,000 readers strong, we know that there is a need and an audience hungry for solid, uplifting, culturally sensitive health information. This book, *Staying Strong: Reclaiming the Wisdom of African-American Healing*, is an extension of the *HealthQuest* mission. It is filled with information that will motivate, inspire, educate and empower. We are thrilled to build on the magazine's legacy by offering a thorough examination of natural healing and what it means for our community.

As the African proverb states, "It takes a village to raise a child." And so it was with producing this book. Many thanks to all of the writers, editors, researchers, visual artists and general supporters who contributed their time, intellect and energy to this collaborative venture. Special thanks to the three principal writers, Kirk Johnson, Egypt Freeman, and Gerda Gallop, and to Dr. Therman Evans, our medical editor.

This book has been touched by many dedicated hands. We hope that it will touch you.

In good health,

SARA LOMAX REESE
Publisher, *HealthQuest* Magazine

Contents

≡ Preface ≡

Congratulations! If you're looking for a surefire way to start getting healthy, staying healthy, and living healthy, you've come to the right place. You're about to learn about Whole Living—a wonderfully exciting tool that every African American can use to achieve unprecedented levels of health, wholeness, and happiness.

This book, *Staying Strong: Reclaiming the Wisdom of African American Healing*, celebrates Whole Living. The book explains how you can use alternatives to mainstream medicine to heal body, mind, and spirit. Many of these alternative healing methods are rooted in respected traditions from Africa, Asia, Europe, and elsewhere, where they have been used with success for centuries. Increasing numbers of African Americans like you are realizing that while modern medicine plays an important role in our lives, doctors don't hold all the answers to what ails us. We're learning that there's a lot to gain by examining alternatives to conventional medicine, discovering the healing traditions of other cultures— and rediscovering our own traditions. Using alternative healing methods connects us "back to our roots," which is a giant step toward Whole Living.

Do you need Whole Living? The answer is yes if you—like all of us at one time or another—have ever felt "stuck" when it comes to thinking about your health. Maybe you're unhappy with the care you're getting from your doctor, but you feel you don't have another alternative.

Maybe you feel so depressed, isolated, or just plain worn out that you want to holler—but you can't figure out why.

Maybe you already take steps to keep yourself healthy and vibrant, and you want to do even more to safeguard your health.

Maybe cancer or heart disease or another major killer of African Americans runs in your family, and you don't know how to stop worrying that it may strike you next.

Maybe you're convinced that as an African American in a hostile world, you've got to look out for number one—if you don't who will? you figure—but it bothers you when folks say you're self-centered.

Maybe you spend a lot of time toning your muscles and building your stamina, but if the truth be known, you still feel your health could be even better.

Maybe you spend so much energy trying to stay one step ahead of your racist (or sexist or homophobic or otherwise intolerant) boss, coworkers, landlord, neighbor, or teacher that you don't have much time to even think about your health.

If you've ever felt that the keys to genuine health and healing seem to lie just beyond your reach, then you need to know about Whole Living. No matter how discouraged you may feel about your physical, emotional, or spiritual health, Whole Living can help you learn to live each moment fully, confidently, and enjoyably.

As you've probably guessed, Whole Living is more than just a different way of thinking about health. It's a revolutionary way of thinking about life. It's a fresh attitude and a revitalizing approach to negotiating your personal journey through life in a way that celebrates the vitality that lives inside of you.

That's why Whole Living is a pathway to health that no African American can afford to ignore.

So what is Whole Living exactly?

In the simplest terms, it's a way of life that celebrates community, commitment, balance, interconnections, and sufficiency. As you read more about Whole Living in the pages ahead, you'll understand these five principles—and more importantly, how you can attain them.

What are other characteristics of Whole Living?

- It's natural. In other words, it works with nature's rhythms, not against them. Whole Living is not about high-tech diagnostic techniques or harsh pharmaceuticals with toxic side effects. It's all about using herbs, touch, foods, and the power of the mind to heal the body and transform the spirit.

- It's spiritual. Your health means more than prescriptions and copayments. It means living life in its fullness, which means nurturing every component—physical, emotional, and certainly spiritual—of who you are. For African Americans, our salvation is—and always has been—our spirit. You can't have genuine health without a vibrant spirit.

- It respects many healing traditions. Modern medicine clearly has an important place for African Americans—why not use every healing tool at our disposal?—but it's only one method. Whole Living uses a combined approach that draws on diverse healing traditions. That way, you get to enjoy richer benefits than any single method can offer.

- It looks at the whole picture. They say the whole is the sum of its parts. But looking at human beings—or anything else, for that matter—as just a bunch of isolated parts isn't very healthy, because everything inside you and around you is interconnected. By Whole Living, you build your health in its entirety.

Those are some of the reasons why *Staying Strong: Reclaiming the Wisdom of African American Healing* is a major departure from other books on Black health. Crack open a typical book on Black health and what do you find? Gloom-and-doom statistics on how such-and-such disease hits our community harder than others. Grim facts and figures about how we don't get Pap smears and prostate examinations as often as we should. Depressing analyses of how Black folks don't have the same access to respectful health care as Whites. It's a pretty disturbing message, when you think about it: we're sick, we don't take care of ourselves, and doctors don't treat us right.

Now, it's true that many of us aren't exactly role models when it comes to caring for ourselves. We hoist ourselves out of bed each morning and tell ourselves, hey, we've done our exercise for the day. Then we sit down to the breakfast table and throw down enough grease to supply an international oil cartel. We fly from task to task, rarely taking a quiet moment to be aware of the world around us. And when something goes wrong, we delay seeing a doctor ("Oh, it'll clear up . . .") until we can barely crawl to the hospital. So it's true: sometimes we bring illness on ourselves.

The medical profession isn't much better. If we're fortunate to have health insurance and access to a doctor's office, we can feel mighty disappointed once we get there. Many doctors don't take the time to appreciate the whole patient, so they can't possibly provide for the whole patient. The quality of care often suffers terribly as a result, especially when the patient has brown skin.

But when we talk about how the health care system doesn't treat us right, it takes attention away from the power we have to heal ourselves.

When we spotlight the ways that the high cost of laboratory tests and prescription medicines puts Black folks at a disadvantage, it distracts us from alternative healing approaches that are usually much more affordable.

Granted, we can all take better care of our health. But focusing on what we fail to do eclipses the more important issue of what we can do. Concentrating on what we *don't* have makes us lose sight of the miraculous capabilities we *do* have.

These are just some of the reasons why the book you're holding could be one of the most important investments you can make in yourself.

You're going to like this book. It's upbeat, because Whole Living helps you move from despair to repair. It helps you appreciate the many reasons to celebrate your health. You should finish this book with a smile on your face—and that good feeling should stay with you long after you've put the book down.

Best of all, it's reader-friendly. No lofty preaching, no complex medical jargon, no hard-to-follow instructions. The emphasis is on simple, specific, step-by-step practical advice you can use immediately.

Part One ("Whole Living") explains how alternative healing methods can help you—and every African American—live a fuller, happier, healthier life.

Chapter 1 ("A History of Healing") introduces you to the history of traditional African healing. African Americans' instinct for healing comes from our history, so to appreciate our "today" we have to understand our "yesterday." Chapter 1 explains how African healing traditions evolved over the centuries, and how they continue to sustain African Americans today. It also explains what the healing traditions of Africa have in common with those of India, China, and other cultures. Whole Living incorporates a variety of healing methods. Once you understand what these many rich traditions have to offer, you'll have a foundation for incorporating them into your life.

Chapter 2 ("Three Health Personalities") suggests that most African Americans think about our health in distinctive ways; you might say we all have a "health personality." This chapter explores three such health personalities: the Sickness Personality, the Wellness Personality, and the Wholeness Personality.

Chapter 3 ("Whole Living—Getting It, Doing It, Loving It")

explains how to identify *your* health personality. Whatever health personality you happen to have—Sickness, Wellness, Wholeness, or somewhere in between—your goal is Wholeness. The closer you come to having a Wholeness Personality, the more you'll be Whole Living. Once you identify your health personality, you can use Chapter 3 to chart your own personal strategy for moving to Wholeness. Your strategy can incorporate alternative healing methods explained in Part II.

Part Two ("Ways to Heal") explores ten alternative healing methods, from acupuncture to vitamin therapy. Each chapter explains how the methods work and the health problems for which they are best suited. They also explain what you should expect from treatment, how much treatment typically costs, and how to find a practitioner (if necessary). You'll also find testimonials from African American healers and patients, to give you a feel for people's actual experiences.

Part Three ("Help Yourself") is all about specific health concerns. If you're looking for advice about a particular condition, whether it be fatigue, heart disease, or any of more than thirty diseases and health problems, including those that affect African Americans disproportionately, you can turn to Part Three for reliable information on alternative approaches. Each entry defines the illness, lists symptoms, and explains what the cause is. You'll read impressive testimonials from African Americans who've used alternative healing approaches successfully to address particular health concerns. Each entry goes on to give advice on specific remedies and advice on prevention.

A final note: you'll meet many new people in this book. A few of them are fictional composites; we've given them initials instead of surnames (for example, John T.). Everyone else is real.

Are you ready to embark on your journey to Wholeness? Terrific! Before you do, grab a pencil and take this brief quiz that will help you identify your health personality.

There are no "right" or "wrong" answers: just try to be as

honest as you can. If your response to a given question doesn't appear among the answers given, choose the answer that best reflects your feelings. Don't worry about scoring just yet; you'll score the quiz and interpret the results in Chapter 3.

Good health and healing to you!

Health Personality Quiz

Answer the following questions as honestly as you can. If none of the answers pertains to you, select the one that comes closest to expressing your feelings or beliefs.

1. When I get sick:
   a. I think about the things I need to help me feel better.
   b. I think about what I have that will help me feel better.
   c. I assume I have everything I need to help me feel better.

2. In general, people would be happier if:
   a. They were less fixated on the past or on the future.
   b. They were more patient and waited for events to unfold.
   c. They had had happier childhoods.

3. When I exercise, I like to:
   a. Develop specific areas of my body.
   b. Use the time to think about problems.
   c. Lose track of time and let the experience flow.

4. When I get sick:
   a. I accept the care of others and look forward to reciprocating.
   b. I try to take care of myself.
   c. I rely on others to take care of me.

5. If I won the lottery today, I would probably:
   a. Buy something I've always dreamed of owning.
   b. Place the winnings in a promising long-term investment.
   c. Save some of the money and spend some.

6. On most days, I feel that I have the energy of:
   a. An eager puppy.
   b. A buzzing insect.
   c. A hibernating bear.

7. When I sustain a physical injury:
   a. I let the injured part heal on its own.
   b. I visualize the healing process.
   c. I stay hopeful for a full recovery.

8. When I think about my dreams for my life:
   a. I'm sure they will come true.
   b. I'd like to think they'll come true.
   c. I doubt that they'll come true.

9. In my home I have:
   a. Few or no photos of my family and close friends.
   b. Some photos of my family and close friends.
   c. Many photos of my family and close friends.

10. If I were hospitalized with an illness or injury, my doctor would probably find me:
    a. Chatting with patients whose spirits need lifting.
    b. Asking questions of the staff and making sure I'm doing everything I can to heal.
    c. Probably a bit disoriented because of the new surroundings.

11. My philosophy is:
    a. You scratch my back first.
    b. A penny saved is a penny earned.
    c. Do unto others as you would have them do unto you.

12. When I'm not feeling well:
    a. I become committed to feeling better.
    b. I get involved in feeling better.
    c. I'm always interested in feeling better.

13. When I catch a cold from someone I know is sick, I feel:
    a. Resentful that they weren't more careful about spreading germs.
    b. Responsible for taking the risk of being near them.
    c. Accountable for my own health and for not spreading the cold to others.

14. If I were stuck in traffic and late for an appointment, and I suddenly saw an opportunity that would save me time but delay other drivers, I would:
    a. Not take it, because the other drivers might be running late, too.
    b. Take it and by my example show other drivers the opportunity, too.
    c. Take it and be grateful that the odds were in my favor.

15. If my doctor told me I needed to change my lifestyle, I would probably think:
    a. It would be a lot easier to take a pill.
    b. I'm willing to change, even if it will only benefit my health in the distant future.
    c. I'm willing to change, especially if it will bring results soon.

16. My ideal health care professional is:
    a. Humble. It shows they're dedicated to their patients, not their egos.
    b. Decisive. It shows they're confident about their work.
    c. Wealthy. It shows they're successful.

17. I get the feeling that people think I need to:
    a. Think less of myself and more of others.
    b. Relax and try to be more impulsive.
    c. Take more credit for my accomplishments.

18. If I visited a health professional because I was having difficulty sleeping at night, I would feel disappointed if he or she didn't:
    a. Discuss my physical, emotional, and spiritual well-being.
    b. Ask me about any physical health problems that may affect my sleep.
    c. Offer to prescribe medicine to help me feel drowsy.

19. I think the most important determinant of my health is:
    a. My genes and my upbringing.
    b. My plans to eat better and exercise more.
    c. What I'm doing today to be healthy.

20. When I'm in a dangerous situation, I think:
    a. Someone who's watching over me will protect me.
    b. I can escape this if I use my wits.
    c. If someone had done their job correctly, this probably wouldn't have happened.

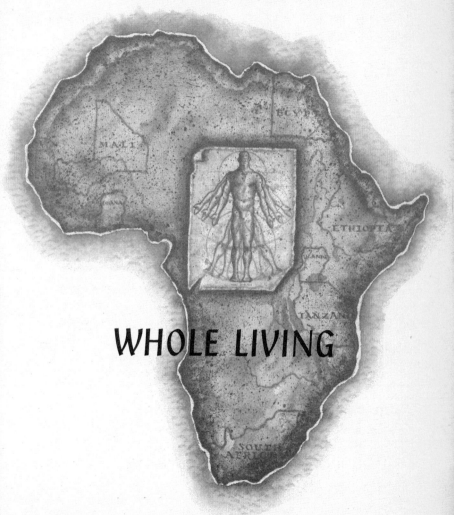

WHOLE LIVING

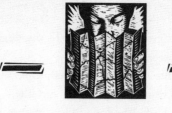

CHAPTER 1

A History of Healing

In a dusty and placid African village, a small boy is on his hands and knees. With handfuls of wet sand he's fashioning a tiny hut, a miniature version of the one he and his family sleep in at night. Moments later, the boy's scream pierces the midday quiet. Transfixed by his construction project, he has backed into the smoldering remnants of the cooking fire. An elder hurries to the boy's side carrying a leaf broken from an aloe plant, a traditional remedy for burns. She smears the plant's thick juice on the toes of the whimpering youngster she cradles in her arms. After a few minutes of reassurance, the boy is giggling once again.

Now come with us to suburban America. On a backyard patio, a chubby kindergartner in pigtails, her cocoa-brown skin already darkening under the early summer sun, "helps" her father barbecue a rack of sizzling chicken breasts. Across the fence, her neighbor is adding a room to his house. Distracted by the sudden screech of a power saw next door, the girl leans too close to the searing-hot grill. The sound of her pain floods the air. Quickly her mother breaks a leaf from the aloe plant on the kitchen windowsill and gently touches the juice to the mark on her daughter's arm. Before long, the carefree youngster is racing off to the sandbox, her sundress waving in the breeze.

These two accounts may be fictional, but they ring true. Through turbulent centuries and across turbulent seas, we have always known how to heal. We don't always realize how we know; we rarely consider why we know: but we know. Call it a sense for healing, an instinct for wellness. It permeates the African American psyche, providing reassurance and comfort since the days when life was more dangerous, and fate more uncertain.

We often think of traditional medicine—anthropologists call it "ethnomedicine" to distinguish it from modern medicine or "biomedicine"—as superstitious, even primitive. But in some ways it's more sophisticated than modern medicine. African-based ethnomedicine takes stock of an ailing person in her or his entirety, restoring health by finding balance within family and community as well as body and spirit. It's an approach that gives fresh new dimensions to how we think about health, offering natural remedies without prescription medicines, supernatural communication without churches, dream testing without psychiatry, health rituals without fitness clubs. And it can be amazingly effective: African healers often achieve stunning results that leave western observers scratching their heads in disbelief.

To understand how these traditional methods work, take a moment to appreciate how Africans view the world. Now, Africa is a land of many peoples, each with their own distinctive cultures and traditions. Historians say that when it comes to healing, Africa has been influenced by war and conquest, and by the migratory ebbs and flows that have commingled Jewish, Greek, Indian, Christian, Moslem, and other traditions with longstanding local cultures. So there's a great deal of diversity on the continent. Even so, many common threads remain—enough of them to weave a composite picture of an African way of healing. It's a way of thinking that's about as different from most Americans' perspectives as, well, Black and White.

The African Worldview

When anthropologists want to study traditional African healers, they load up the Jeep, hire a driver, and head for the African countryside, where time-honored ways of life remain largely unchanged by the rest of the world's rush to be modern. A recent report from the bush illustrates several distinctive features of ethnomedical healing.

In a South African village near the city of Empangeni, a village leader was ailing. He was terribly depressed, too, because he couldn't shake a recent string of bad luck. A traditional healer—a diviner—who was called to the scene knew just what to do. The diviner recalls, "The first night at Empangeni, my grandfather's spirit appeared and informed me that the head of this village was no longer visited by his ancestors. This is why he was sick and unlucky."

The healer prayed to the man's ancestors on his behalf and gave him an herbal potion to make him vomit. Then he sacrificed a white hen. "Actually, the ancestors had called for a white cock," the diviner explained, "but since we could not find one, we placed twenty cents on the sacrifice to make it acceptable."

Ancestor worship? Ritual sacrifice? It may sound awfully primitive—even embarrassing—for those of us whose impressions of Africans have been forged by those degrading Tarzan movies. But strip away Hollywood's warped lens and the countless other racist distortions of Africans that confront us from birth, and you'll find a healing tradition whose longevity is a testament to its value.

In fact, ethnomedicine remains immensely popular in South Africa. Eighty percent of the population consults the estimated

300,000 traditional healers, accounting for an astounding 100 million visits each year. Unlike during the apartheid era when the White South African government dismissed traditional healing as pure fantasy, the nation's new leaders recognize the value of traditional medicine, or *muti*. Today officials are starting to subject traditional cures to scientific tests. "For despite the 'mumbo-jumbo' there is little doubt that some *muti* works," reports the southern Africa newspaper, *The Independent*.

African ethnomedicine embraces a worldview of interconnectedness. Traditional African culture emphasizes the interconnections between families, neighbors, coworkers, and ancestors in a vast continuum that also includes God, powerful spirits, and inanimate objects. In an ideal cosmos, these many entities would coexist in harmony. But life is never ideal. Just like everyone else, Africans get sick, they have accidents, they get fired from their jobs, their cars break down. And so when illness or other misfortune strikes, Africans view it as discord in the cosmos. The source of the discord might be a disease-carrying insect, or punishment by God or an ancestor for someone's wrongdoing, or even a hex inflicted by an envious or spiteful troublemaker. Any way you slice it, the result is bad fortune. The aim in ethnomedicine is to figure out who or what is responsible for the imbalance that's causing trouble, and to restore harmony.

The interconnectedness of the elements in the African cosmos means that Africans view the world with a profound unity. There are few clear distinctions between the natural and the supernatural, or dreams and reality. The mind and body aren't separate: they flow through each other, allowing mental illness to be treated with a physical therapy or vice versa. Life and time are one, a concept that enables the living to communicate with long-deceased ancestors, whom Africans consider frightfully powerful and very nearly omniscient, although approachable by the living. It was natural, then, for the South African diviner to commune with his dead grandfather's spirit and for him to pray to the village leader's ancestors. He was consulting a higher authority for direction, then following through with the prescription.

Unlike many physicians, who merely try to understand what is wrong with a patient, traditional African healers help patients understand why they are afflicted and who is responsible. This reflects the African view that illness is linked not just to cause but to motivation and a responsible party. In Empangeni, the diviner determined that the ancestors of the village head were no longer visiting him. Having ascertained the "why" of the illness, he could then offer a remedy.

African remedies also blend religion and science. They might involve ritual, communication with ancestors, avoidance of something considered spirit-possessed, or treatment with a remedy derived from plant, mineral, or animal products. The herbs that caused vomiting in the Empangeni case are a common form of treatment. The intent is to purge the body of the evil placed there, in this case, by a displeased ancestor.

And finally, traditional African healing is characterized by exceptional openness. When the Empangeni diviner improvised to create the sacrificial equivalent of a white rooster, he added to a long tradition of flexibility. It's not uncommon in modern Africa to find the curious sight of traditional herbalists who use stethoscopes, and diviners who pore over psychotherapy textbooks. People use whatever works. This openness means the traditional methods of African healing can adapt to the demands of a changing world. Considering the history of African healing, this flexibility has surely ensured its resilience.

African Healing in Antiquity

The Empangeni case shows that much of African ethnomedicine is rooted in the belief in magic and spirits. That's because religion lies at the core of African life. "It is no exaggeration," suggests Kofi Asare Opoku, author of *West African Traditional Religion* (FEP International, 1978), "to say that in traditional Africa, religion is life, and life, religion." Early Africans, seeking an explanation for their baffling shifts of fortune—good health, a successful birth, or bountiful harvest one year, sickness, barrenness, or drought the next—reasoned that the universe was under divine control. Because they had little power to affect the course of daily events, they figured that contacting this divinity would help them avoid misfortune. Thus were born the first diviners, practitioners of a magical art that by one estimate dates to 4000 B.C. Diviners flourished in Babylonia and ancient Egypt, where they were called to analyze dreams, interpret celestial movements, and decipher sacrificial entrails.

Diviners, later known as medicine men, witchdoctors, or root doctors, frequently complemented supernatural interpretations by prescribing plant- and animal-based remedies. Many of these, too, were based on magic: a lion's heart was believed useful for imparting strength, a tortoiseshell extract was given to help a person be resilient. This strategy—divination for diagnosis, natural remedies for treatment—established a model for centuries to come. Sorcerers and witches practiced a second tradition. These evil-doers practiced negative medicine—black magic, ritual murder—and were universally feared. Over the years, Africa was also influenced by Islamic medicine, which weds Greek, Iranian, Indian, and other principles of diet, health, and views of humankind's relationship with the world.

Not many people realize it, but Africa also has a long tradition of scientific medicine. In fact, scholars trace the roots of biomedicine not to Rome or Greece, but to ancient Egypt. The first physician known to history by name may have been Athonis, who ruled Egypt for twenty-seven years as its second king around 3200 B.C., and who is said to have written detailed anatomy books. Another leading physician was named Imhotep. This multitalented archi-

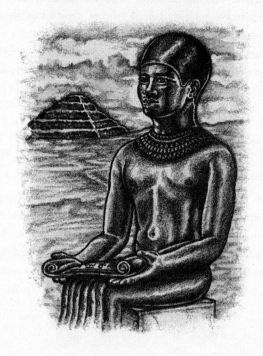

tect, scribe, priest, administrator, and member of pharoah's court lived around 2980 B.C. Imhotep was such an extraordinarily skilled physician that within 100 years of his death he was elevated to the status of deity—a feat never before attained by a mortal in Egyptian history, according to Charles S. Finch, Ph.D., author of *The African Background to Medical Science* (Karnak House, 1990). "Hippocrates may be widely known as the 'Father of Medicine'," says Finch, but "if such a title belongs to anyone, it belongs to Imhotep."

These and other African healers compiled remarkably detailed information about physical diagnosis, pathology, and herbal pharmacology. One collection of papyrus records, called the Ebers Papyrus (1500 B.C.), contains chapters on dermatology, ophthalmology, intestinal disease, contraception, obstetrics and gynecology, dentistry, and the surgical treatment of abscesses, tumors, burns, and fractures. Egyptian papyri from 2500 to 300 B.C. show pictographs of needles and ingenious absorbable suture material braided from animal gut—the same stuff surgeons use today.

From these earliest days, Africans developed and refined over ensuing generations their diverse healing traditions into a coherent and trusted body of knowledge. These traditions include belief in:

- God, the creator of the world and source of all power—"the one beyond all thanks," as some Africans put it—who both rewards the living for their goodness and punishes them for their misdeeds;

- ancestral spirits—powerful deceased relatives who are believed to maintain a presence among the living ("like a cloud of witnesses," according to anthropologist Geoffrey Parrinder), and who, like God, punish and reward the living (though always for just cause) and are consulted by the living in times of need;

- in some societies, nature gods—lesser deities associated with rivers, rocks, or other elements of the natural world;

- in some societies, certain plants and animals viewed as sacred emblems that once played a crucial role in the survival of forebears;

- witches (malevolent people who can hurt others simply by thinking them harm) and sorcerors (who can harness nature's forces—rain, lightning, drought, disease—for evil purposes). Witches and sorcerors are the African equivalent of Christianity's devil; they're the "demonic humanity" that are the root of all evil, says B.C. Ray, author of *African Religions: Symbol, Ritual, and Community* (Prentice-Hall, 1976).

- herbalists, diviners, root doctors, and medicine men and women. These healers practice magic to harness nature's forces. Unlike witchcraft or sorcery, which is always destructive, magic can be used for both positive and negative purposes. Constructively, a diviner or root doctor might use ritual and an herbal mixture to heal the sick. Destructively, they might "put a root" on an unfortunate victim, often at the request of a malicious person who, because of jealousy, spitefulness, or revenge, wishes the victim harm.

- charms, amulets, and talismans, which are used both protectively and offensively.

You can see already that African ethnomedicine is complex stuff. Forget the stereotypes: there's nothing simplistic about this sophisticated healing art.

And there's more. In addition to these magical and religious traditions, Africans collected a vast storehouse of knowledge about native plants. How vast? When two researchers from South Africa's University of the Witwatersrand in Johannesburg, South Africa, decided in the early 1920s to compile a book of medicinal and poisonous plants used in southern and eastern Africa alone, they devoted forty years to the project, eventually cataloguing some 11,000 separate plant items.

So when twenty Africans disembarked at Jamestown, Virginia, in 1619, they and the hundreds of thousands of slaves who followed them carried rich, bountiful healing traditions that were thousands of years old. In America these venerated traditions would do more than simply keep us healthy. They would help ensure our very survival.

Traditional Healing During Slavery

The ships that brought slaves to the New World also brought plants. Some of these—okra, yams, black-eyed peas—went to the dinner table. Others joined new medicinal plants that slaves discovered through contact with Native Americans or by trial-and-error experimentation. The result was a new medicine chest of herbal cures. This ingenuity would serve slaves well, because sickness loomed large in the days of slavery. Health was precarious for both Whites and Blacks but it was enslaved Africans, who sometimes subsisted on marginal diets and slept in leaky, drafty housing with primitive sanitation, who were at particular risk. Yellow fever, cholera, typhoid, and malaria wiped out thousands.

In the face of such misery, slaves were often prohibited from practicing traditional healing methods. Historians cite two reasons. Slaves' extensive knowledge of herbal poisons greatly alarmed Whites, who feared deadly retribution from their chattel. Whites also feared that Blacks, traveling from one plantation to another under the guise of practicing medicine, might convey intelligence about plans for a slave revolt. So the courts outlawed the practice of ethnomedicine, sometimes under penalty of death.

Yet slaves never wavered in their devotion to traditional methods. For hundreds of years they quietly continued to patronize respected Black healers. Some Whites did, too. Midwives and herbalists covertly engaged in healing rituals, used an array of plant remedies to mend the sick, and fashioned charms to protect themselves from sorcery. Why, you might ask, would anyone risk death for a good-luck charm or a handful of herbs?

Well, there are lots of reasons. For one, until about 1900 the practice of biomedicine—what we now know as modern medicine—was pretty primitive. For instance, many doctors mistakenly believed that disease was caused by an imbalance of body humors such as blood and bile, or by odors given off by decaying animal and vegetable matter. Thus, malaria was thought to be caused not by the bite of a parasite-infected mosquito, but by what one physician called "most noxious exhalations" from swamps.

What's more, the typical treatment for malaria and other illnesses was no picnic. To rid the body of accumulated poisons, doctors bled patients by pushing small spring-loaded knives into the skin, or by applying blood-sucking leaches, sometimes until the patient fainted. Other cleansing tactics induced sweating, skin blistering, or vomiting. These treatments frequently failed. "The poor negroes, treated like white men, continued to get sick and die," wrote Dr. Samuel Cartwright in 1854 in reference to a dysentery outbreak on a Louisiana plantation.

That's not to say that slaves' own remedies were flawless—they weren't. In 1800, Thomas Jefferson's daughter Martha wrote to her father about a slave named Jupiter who, believing himself poisoned, consulted a Black healer who administered medicine he said would either kill or cure. The patient fell into convulsions and died, after which the doctor fled.

But slaves' remedies were not only much gentler than those of their owners, but in some cases remarkably effective. "The old folks knowed lots of ways to cure things," recalled ex-slave Janey Landrum.

Take the case of Jack, a Black man owned by Virginia planter John Walker. In the summer of 1833, Walker wrote in his diary that Jack had developed an alarming eye affliction. A White doctor treated Jack for an entire month, but the slave's vision only declined further. On 5 June 1833, Walker sent Jack to, in the farmer's imperfect grammar, "and Old Negro Man Named Lewis who says he can cure him." When the slave returned to the planter on 19 July, the transformation was miraculous. "Jack went over to him . . . almost blind," Walker wrote in amazement. "His sight seems as good as ever." It was the same story in Tennessee in 1844, where a slaveowner indicted for allowing his slave to practice traditional medicine told the court that the "obedient, exemplary slave . . . had performed many cures of a most extraordinary nature."

But to understand the entire appeal of traditional slave remedies, you have to understand their influence on the body and the spirit. Like their African ancestors, slaves lived in a world of heightened spirituality where deceased relatives, diverse spirits, and magical spells from sorcerors exerted a powerful influence over day-to-day life. This spiritual element, which was absent from biomedicine, was an important part of their ethnomedicine.

Listen to former slave Della Barksdale, whose infant was so sick with bronchitis that a doctor had given up hope. Suddenly, she recalled to an interviewer, the spirit of her deceased mother appeared and instructed her to mix lard and quinine into a salve for the baby. She did, and the remedy brought immediate relief. When the doctor returned, he was incredulous. "What on earth did you do?" he asked. Recalls Barksdale, "I tole him 'twont my business to tell him, 'twas his business to tell me."

The spiritual dimension of the traditional African worldview gave slaves a degree of mental control not only over their health, but over the brutality of slavery as well. In a world where the next bend in the road could bring arbitrary cruelty, belief in magic helped slaves feel that they could influence their own fate, which helped them preserve their sanity. A slave might interpret the song of a certain bird or the twitch of an eye as a warning sign, and maneuver successfully to avoid being whipped. "No doubt chance, hard work, or good behavior coincided with magic to stave off beatings," suggests historian Elliott Gorn, Ph.D. "But conjuring allowed slaves to believe they manipulated whites."

Magic served other important functions, too. It gave slaves a source of information and a body of knowledge that was removed from Whites' control because it was centered squarely in the Black community and in African traditions. Anthropologist Holly F. Mathews, Ph.D., of East Carolina University, says this unifying influence of magic, which drew together enslaved Africans from diverse tribes and cultural backgrounds, gave slaves strength. "It is not surprising that magic helped give many slaves the courage to persevere and even to rebel against their oppressors," she writes in *Herbal and Magical Medicine* (Duke University Press, 1993).

Finally, magic maintained order in the slave community. For instance, slaves didn't think twice about stealing from their owners. "Their logic was impeccable," says historian Eugene D. Genovese, Ph.D., author of *Roll, Jordan, Roll* (Pantheon Books, 1974). "If they belonged to their masters, how could they steal from him?" Slaves figured that eating one of their owner's chickens or some of his corn only transformed his property from one form into another, much as they did when they fed the corn to the chickens. But stealing from another slave was a different story altogether, because retribution in the form of a magical spell could be swift and unmerciful. Thus, belief in people's ability to harness the power of the world around them and inflict injury on others provided welcome order in otherwise difficult and unpredictable lives.

So ethnomedicine offered slaves important elements of safety and security as well as healing. Over the years, slaves' ethnomedical traditions evolved; to the vast collection of beliefs and practices they carried from Africa, slaves not only added Native Americans' extensive knowledge of plant cures but even borrowed Europeans' practice of purging and bleeding the sick. Eventually, the formal practice of ethnomedicine went further underground (although many continued the practice in private), as Black converts to Protestantism proclaimed sorcery and magic to be the works of the devil. But no matter. Regardless of its form, and irrespective of mainstream opinion, ethnomedicine endured. And it did so largely because of one essential truth: by providing useful remedies in times of illness, plus vital protection for the psyche, it gave Black folks who labored in a hostile world a measure of comfort and reassurance that was in short supply.

African Healing After Slavery

The Civil War era was a turning point for biomedicine. Before 1850 or so, doctoring was a hit-and-miss affair. Sally Brown, an 89-year-old ex-slave from Georgia, explained that when a doctor visited the sick, "He'd try one medicine and if it didn't do no good he'd try another." But the next fifty years brought an astonishing number of medical developments. The stethoscope was invented in 1851, allowing doctors a noninvasive window inside their patients. In 1867, the use of disinfectants permitted clean surgery and shattered doctors' belief that infection was a natural stage of healing. In the 1870s, the thermometer came into popular use, allowing doctors to replace an instrument so bulky that it had to be carried under one arm.

Suddenly medical examinations were easier, diagnosis was more accurate, drugs were more effective, and surgery was safer. You'd think it was the perfect prescription for Black folks.

But medical advances are one thing; access to them is another. While the plantation system gave slave owners a reason to provide doctors for slaves as a way to maintain the system's labor-power, newly freed slaves were poor—too poor to afford private doctors' fees. Not that Blacks who could pay were particularly welcome in the health care system in the first place. Many White-controlled hospitals refused outright to admit Blacks. And freedmen who were fortunate enough to locate a more liberal-minded hospital found themselves on segregated wards with brutally disrespectful standards of care. Throughout the nineteenth century, Black patients had been subjected to rude pokings and proddings by eager medical students; others were singled out to demonstrate surgical techniques. "On these all-Black wards, it wasn't uncommon for a White doctor to ask medical students if they had ever seen an amputation," says medical historian W. Michael Byrd, M.D., M.P.H., of the Harvard School of Public Health. "If they hadn't, the doctor would randomly select a Black patient and amputate a perfectly healthy leg on the spot."

That may sound inconceivable given the respectful treatment many hospitals provide today. But a century ago, racist interpretations of physiological and intellectual differences between Whites and Blacks melded with the Darwinian theory of survival of the fittest and convinced many Whites that Negroes were a vastly inferior subspecies. White doctors were no exception. Dr. Samuel Cartwright, a prominent southern surgeon, articulated the popular view, speculating that "a deficiency of cerebral matter in the cranium" had "rendered the people of Africa unable to take care of themselves."

This presumption of racial superiority opened the door to more than the violation of the living. Medical school instructors who needed cadavers for human dissection headed straight for African Americans, a vulnerable population that was powerless to resist. Hurried dissections of Blacks before a family could claim a body were common, as was grave-robbing.

So there were plenty of reasons not to trust the White medical establishment. Why not turn to African American physicians— professionals we could count on to provide respectful care? Well, easier said than done. Black students were systematically denied entry into medical schools in the United States until the 1840s. So for many decades, there weren't a lot of Black doctors to go around. As late as 1920, there were just five Black physicians in the entire city of Detroit, Michigan.

When Black doctors did emerge from medical training and tried to establish their practices, they mostly met hostility from their White colleagues. Whites denied Black doctors admitting privileges at hospitals, thereby forcing them into the humiliating and financially costly position of handing over their patients to White doctors. African Americans were barred from joining the American Medical Association from 1869—when three prestigious Black physicians in Washington, D.C., applied unsuccessfully for membership—until the civil rights movement of the 1960s. In 1895, Black doctors responded by organizing their own group— the National Medical Association—a Washington, D.C.-based organization that's still up and running, 14,500 members strong.

So African Americans emerging from the Civil War years faced a dilemma. Biomedicine was maturing in leaps and bounds, but access to its remedies was severely limited for Black folks, and we couldn't be sure of decent care if we found a doctor who would treat us. Under the circumstances, why not turn to Miss Lydia, the gray-haired widow down the road, the one they say knows every herb in the woods? Why not head over to see Sister Susie, the midwife who's got so many successful birthings under her belt that she's lost count of them all? Why not ask Uncle Joe, the fellow who stepped in last year after the doctors gave up on that young woman in the next county, and who saved her from the root (hex) someone had put on her?

Is it any mystery that by 1930, there were an estimated 5,000 Black midwives, each of them "catching" babies and dispensing soul-comforting folk remedies, in Virginia alone? Or that an Alabama physician, baffled but impressed by his patients' persistent belief in voodoo, would write in a medical journal, "So firm is this belief that no sort of reason will shake it"?

The fact is, during Reconstruction and beyond, Black folks turned to ethnomedicine for many of the same reasons that we did so earlier—for effectiveness and reassurance. And now there was a new incentive, a financial one. For people who had to shell out payment for their own care, it made perfect sense to patronize a herbalist or a root doctor rather than risking the high cost of visiting a White physician—a doctor who might treat you badly on top of that.

Black Healing in Modern Times

They say the more things change, the more they remain the same. That's a good way to think about Black health, because many of the currents that sweep African Americans toward the new millennium are really the same waters we've traveled for centuries now.

Case in point: the Tuskegee experiment. In 1932 when U.S. Public Health Service physicians promised 431 syphilitic Black men in Tuskegee, Alabama, treatment for their "bad blood," none of the men could have possibly guessed that the medicine they would receive was actually nothing more than aspirin and vitamins. For the idea wasn't to treat the men at all, but—in a malignant perversion of scientific curiosity—to observe untreated syphilis as it slowly killed them. And kill them it did, one by one.

When the experiment began, syphilis was an incurable disease that ravaged its victims, often causing crippling or fatal nerve damage. By the mid-1940s, however, researchers had discovered a cure—a simple two-week course of penicillin. And still the Tuskegee study continued. Only when a reporter blew the whistle in 1972 did a chastened Uncle Sam, embarrassed by the national outrage over the scandal, shut the study down. By then, all but a handful of the poor, uneducated sharecroppers in the study, had died, their families collecting $50 in "burial insurance"—$35 for the families, $15 for the undertaker—that had helped secure the men's participation. And it wasn't until 1997 that President Bill Clinton offered a formal apology on behalf of the federal government.

Appalling and shameful as it is, there's nothing particularly new about Tuskegee. By the time federal researchers had decided on this rural farming community as the site for the syphilis study, White doctors had been experimenting on Black folks for decades. We must have appeared to be brown-skinned guinea pigs to the South Carolina physician who in 1838, eager to test his experimental remedies, took newspaper ads offering "the highest cash price" for fifty chronically diseased Negroes whom owners might want to "dispose of." Some White doctors even got rich by experimenting on us. When slave John Brown was given to a physician in gratitude for the doctor's services, the man of medicine realized he had an ideal means to test remedies for heatstroke. Over a period of weeks, he repeatedly forced Brown to sit buried in an oven-like pit until the slave fainted. Then the good doctor proceeded to package what he called medicine for heatstroke—pills containing nothing more than flour and cayenne pepper—with which the physician made what Brown termed "a large fortune."

Just as these horrific abuses made the Black community wary of the biomedical establishment throughout the nineteenth century, Tuskegee's reverberations continue to rumble through the Black community today, some twenty-five years after the study was halted. For example, researchers find they can't recruit Blacks into studies to test new drugs for acquired immune deficiency syndrome (AIDS). The sad irony, of course, is that our community is hit disproportionately hard by the disease. As one physician explained to *Essence* magazine, "Although everyone may not know the specifics of the Tuskegee experiment, they have enough residual knowledge of it so that they mistrust government-sponsored programs, and this results in a lack of participation in [AIDS] risk-reduction efforts." It's much the same story at Los Angeles's Charles Drew University School of Medicine and Science, a historically Black institution, where researchers discovered men who expressed reluctance about participating in prostate cancer research unless they felt they could trust their doctors. Why? The "Syphilis Thing," the men said.

More déjà vu: take a close look at America's two-tiered health care system—private doctors dispensing lavish care on the elite who have health insurance; crumbling public facilities that provide spartan care for the more than 40 million of us who are uninsured or underinsured. This two-tiered system originated over 100 years ago. During Reconstruction, when Jim Crow legislation segregated the nation right down to its water fountains, medical facilities followed suit. There were all-White hospitals and all-Black hospitals; all-White wards, all-Black ones. And despite the heroic work of Black health professionals, the Black facilities, with their uncertain funding and weak political support, invariably had to work harder to stay afloat.

We see the same struggle today in many inner-city and isolated rural health care facilities that serve African Americans. Now that segregation is history, many historically Black hospitals have closed their doors. Of the 400 such hospitals that have existed at one time or another in our nation's history, only about two dozen are still in business. Perennial funding cuts and staff reductions at the few remaining Black hospitals and at the many integrated clinics and hospitals across the land mean that patients, who are often desperately ill, arrive at a health care facility that is struggling to do much more with much less, and where years of high-stress doctoring can leave staff members disheartened, disillusioned, and bitter. Dr. Margaret Heagerty, Director of Pediatrics at Harlem Hospital, New York, says that when patients step through the door of public hospitals, they come face to face with institutions that are designed more for the comfort of the people who provide services than those who receive them. "All of us in the trenches of medical care for the poor can tell war stories about this type of institutional ineptitude and callousness," says Heagerty, writing in the *Journal of Health Care for the Poor and Underserved.* "Block appointments, long waiting times at clinics, lack of interpreters for Spanish-speaking patients, and perhaps most serious, an attitude that is more than a little authoritarian, combining a mixture of colonialism and punitiveness."

Given the choice, once again, between an indifferent if not hostile biomedical health care system and the welcoming, protective embrace of ethnomedicine, you can see why millions of African Americans feel that our African-based health traditions make just as much sense today as they did back at Jamestown in 1619. No wonder anthropologists find bountiful examples of herbal medicine, healing rituals, and other ethnomedical practices from New England to the West Coast, throughout the urban north, and across the rural and urban south. "It is found wherever large numbers of Black people live," says anthropologist Loudell F. Snow, Ph.D., of Michigan State University.

These ethnomedical practices take a variety of forms, some of them sensible, others perhaps less so, but all of them reflecting ingenuity and diligence in a search for healing that transcends the limitations and disappointments of biomedicine. The core of these practices is the belief that healing is larger than the mere exchange of dollars for pills. Genuine healing connects us with ways of living that resonate with those who have walked before us, and in a way that's larger than any of us.

You can see it in Willa Johnson, a forty-year-old professor at the University of Illinois. Johnson enlists several trusted physicians to help bring healing and wholeness to her life, but she also uses a variety of alternative methods. To soothe her soul from the stressful demands of teaching, counseling students, and conducting scholarly research, she practices biofeedback to bathe her inner self with messages of calm. Occasionally she might pour a cup of almond herbal tea or take a homeopathic preparation made from the flowers of impatiens and other plants known to have calming properties. She's big on exercise, too. It gives her strength, endurance, and peace of mind. "The first time I walked on a treadmill, I was so exhausted after two minutes that I thought the trainer was trying to kill me," Johnson says with a smile as she relaxes in her book-lined office. "Last week I ran my first five-mile race, and it was a piece of cake."

But one of Johnson's most enduring comforts is her special relationship with her mother, who died unexpectedly during open-heart surgery when Johnson was just seventeen. Johnson was looking forward to the vacation her mother had promised to take with her on her mother's release from the hospital. She never made it out. "My mother was my very best friend. Not a day goes by without me feeling her presence around me," says Johnson, whose youthful face and close-cropped curls might have earned her a career in modeling. "Every time I achieve a milestone in my personal or professional life, I feel her feeling proud of me."

Unlike Africans, who believe ancestors can inflict illness on the living to punish improper behavior, Johnson doesn't think her mother would ever make her sick. But otherwise, her conception of her mother fits closely with the traditional African notion that our departed ancestors remain with us as a continuing presence. They watch over us, providing comfort, guidance, and soul-healing reassurance.

You can see the healing in Pilar Jan Penn, a thirty-something African American mother, lawyer, and community health advocate in Stone Mountain, Georgia, who, after some fifteen years of studying and living traditional African-centered ways, says her life actually transcends sickness. "Sickness isn't a part of what I do," she says simply. A contented vegetarian, Penn lives a life of mindful spirituality that combines respect for her ancestors with a heightened awareness of her responsibilities to herself and others. On the altars that grace her home lay remembrances of her heritage and her humanity: pictures of her ancestors; a photo of her daughter; seashells; rocks; dried flowers; bowls of water; white, yellow, and green candles; a crystal she discovered in her yard; a piece of wood taken from her grandfather's house. They are artifacts from the earth, reminders of the Middle Passage, representations of her past, present, and future.

"I perform rituals, burn candles, and pray at my altars," says Penn, her face framed with a hundred golden-brown dreadlocks. She's discovered that when you bring spirituality into your daily life, you can perform mundane daily acts—cooking, cleaning, bathings—with reverence, as if they were spiritual acts. And the spiritual acts become habits—things you do daily without putting a lot of thought into it. "I say prayers, pour libations, or light candles as naturally as you brush your teeth or groom your hair," she says.

Yoga plays an important role in Penn's life, as do nature's herbs. When her three-year-old daughter Chisama Ku came down with chickenpox, Penn sought the guidance of neighborhood healers in fashioning a homemade remedy. She mixed oatmeal (a drying agent) and bentonite clay (to draw out toxins) with goldenseal, myrrh, rosemary oil, and other herbs in a combination designed to help build the immune system and cleanse the blood as well as to promote healing of the sores. When she applied the aromatic paste to the skin sores on her daughter, who was squirming in itchy discomfort, the relief was immediate. "She was so happy," Penn recalls. "Her entire body just relaxed, and it gave her the peace that allowed her to fall asleep."

You can even see the healing in the waiting room of Reverend Doctor Rollins, a self-styled "voodoo priest" who works out of his well-kept home in a dreary section of Pontiac, Michigan. His waiting room is packed with clients. They pass the time while waiting by describing their delight over how Rollins has helped them remedy their physical complaints, resolve marital problems, or find a winning number. Each time they discuss their health concerns, they compare the wondrous results they've achieved under Rollins with the failure of their physicians. Like Africans who feel a heart-to-heart connection with a native healer, these African Americans feel they've finally found someone who understands them.

Mr. Johnson, a middle-aged client of Dr. Rollins who has driven fifteen miles from Flint for help with his hypertension, tells Professor Loudell Snow that he would have used dandelion tea for his "pressure" had he been back in his native Mississippi. He has a physician, but he hasn't seen him in over a year. Mr. Johnson doesn't dislike his doctor; he just doesn't have much faith in the doctor's medicine. "If it was any good it would cure you!" he explains. In the waiting room, heads nod in agreement. People seem to have much more faith in the herbal and other natural remedies Rollins prescribes. Later Snow asks Rollins for a natural remedy for hypertension. Rollins recommends swallowing an egg white sprinkled with salt for nine days. Really high blood pressure can be tamed in 15 minutes, he says, by eating a raw egg yolk mixed with a tablespoon of salt.

Tapping Our Mind Power

From a contented professor to a spirit-mindful mother to a voodoo priest: these three vignettes also highlight the need to approach any healing system with intelligent caution. For example, Reverend Doctor Rollins may be free and easy with the salt shaker, but any physician will tell you that all that sodium—with or without the egg—is the very worst thing a hypertensive person could introduce into their system.

At the same time, scientists tell us that the mind has extraordinary influence over the body. Research suggests that people who are content and well adjusted have a much better chance of maintaining their physical health than if they're chronically depressed, angry, or anxious. "We know that in the healing process of anything from an ulcer to diabetes to asthma, the mind is very intricately involved with whether the patient gets better or worse," former Texas health commissioner David Smith, M.D., author of *Healing and the Mind* (Doubleday, 1993), explained to journalist Bill Moyers. When you think about Rev. Dr. Rollins's salt remedy, maybe what counts isn't so much what's in the spoon, but what's in the heart: whether the patient feels understood, provided for, cared about; whether the healing system resonates with the patient's beliefs and needs; whether the patient senses that the remedy just feels right.

The mind-body connection isn't really all that new. Galen, one of the best-known early Greek physicians, observed that women who were full of melancholy seemed to risk a higher chance of developing breast cancer than did happier women. China's most respected ancient medical text, the *Yellow Emperor's Classic of Internal Medicine,* associated each of seven major organs with an emotion: the lungs with grief; the heart with joy; the liver with anger, and so on. The book goes on to show, for example, that too much (or too little) grief might give rise to certain lung ailments.

Our own African traditions provide abundant evidence for the mind-over-body link. Hexing is a prime example. Take the case of Mrs. E., a forty-three-year-old African American woman from rural Virginia, who appeared at a hospital emergency room complaining of abdominal pain. Doctors were mystified; they couldn't find anything wrong with her. But Mrs. E. said she knew what the problem was. She had snakes and spiders crawling inside of her, she said. (Some believers in ethnomedicine fear having animals magically introduced into their bodies—or worse, being turned into an animal.) Mrs. E. and her family and friends were convinced she had been hexed, a suspicion that was confirmed when she visited a root doctor who predicted she would die like a dog. Soon thereafter, the woman began to bark and crawl on all fours. She began to lose her hair and she slept curled up on the floor. On the very morning she was to visit a Philadelphia, Pennsylvania, root doctor to have her hex removed, Mrs. E. died alone in her trailer home.

"This history of hexing is not a unique clinical occurrence," write anthropologist Marilyn K. Nations, Ph.D., and colleagues at the University of Virginia. The fact is, medical journals are bursting with reports of patients who arrive at a hospital with a problem that perplexed doctors can't tie to a cause: pain but no injury, paralysis but no stroke, depression but no tragic life event. These cases sometimes end in tragedy as the patient deteriorates and dies, while surrounded by the most technologically advanced machinery modern medicine has to offer.

That's the power of the mind over the body. Aunt Ferebe Rogers knew all about the importance of the mind in "conjuring," as she called it. Rogers, a former slave from Georgia, recalled an occasion when a conjuror had tried unsuccessfully to influence her. "He try his bes' to overcome me . . . After dat, he tole my husband he couldn't do nuttin' to me, 'cause I didn't believe in him, and dem cunjur-folks can't hurt you less'n you believes in 'em."

Of course, there are many dozens, if not hundreds, of traditional folk remedies that have nothing to do with the mind. Black folks take catnip tea for colic, chamomile for fever, greens for high blood pressure, sassafras as a tonic, and garlic tablets to purify the blood. Some Black mothers use petroleum jelly and witch hazel ointment for diaper rash, or ice-water-and-vinegar douches as a contraceptive: ice water to "slow down the sperm," the vinegar (hopefully) to kill it. These and countless other traditional cures have passed from grandmother to mother to daughter, nurturing each generation with wisdom. Just as the original Jamestown Africans set about identifying helpful plants and minerals in their new environment, these modern-day remedies reflect our community's ability to find valuable treasures in otherwise mundane surroundings—like spotting vitamin-rich dandelion in an overgrown city lot—and to make do with what we have. As one herbal healer said to Professor Loudell Snow, "There's so many vitamins out there that we're walkin' over."

But the fact that many African Americans still do believe in magical medicine also reminds us that ethnomedicine comes from a continent where the mind and the body intertwine, a place where the spiritual and the physical, the natural and the supernatural merge as one. It's a way of thinking our ancestors knew 4,000 years ago—and, ironically, modern scientists are just beginning to endorse.

Science Climbs on Board

As it turns out, modern science is lending support to the nonmagical aspects of ethnomedicine, too. Ethnopharmacologists—scientists who study the uses of plant and mineral remedies in indigenous cultures—say that whether you're walking Africa's tropical forests, trekking across its grasslands, or traversing the continent's mountains, you find traditional remedies that are often remarkably effective.

- Item: When scientists at Institut d'Hygiene in Togo, West Africa, tested eight medicinal plants traditionally used against malaria, they found that all eight inhibited test tube growth of the one-celled Plasmodium organism that causes the disease. In fact, five of the eight were up to 100 percent effective. Malaria, the world's most common tropical disease, affects millions. Its resurgence in recent years, the result of drug-resistant strains of Plasmodium and pesticide-resistant mosquitoes that carry it, suggests that effective plant remedies might be a worthwhile alternative to drug therapy.

- Item: A Nigerian clay called eko, consumed locally for intestinal disorders, is strikingly similar to the active ingredient—also a clay—in the antidiarrheal medicine Kaopectate. According to geologists at Louisiana State University, the clay particles act as microscopic sponges, attracting toxins and bacteria to their surface and reportedly forming a protective coat on the digestive lining. This may explain the custom of "geophagy" (dirt-eating) that's widespread in tropical West Africa, especially among pregnant women, and is not uncommon among African Americans in the South.

- Item: In Nigeria, cancer patients who consult local healers are typically given stew or tea made from the rootbark of Annona senegalensis, a tree that offers a variety of medicinal uses throughout the continent. When curious surgeons from University College Hospital in Ibadan tested extracts of Annona, they found significant anticancer properties and no side effects—a claim yet to be matched by modern chemotherapy, which can be effective but debilitating. Traditional medicine gets a bad rap from people who complain that it's unscientific, writes Dr. J.I. Durodola, who carried out the study. But, he says, the fact

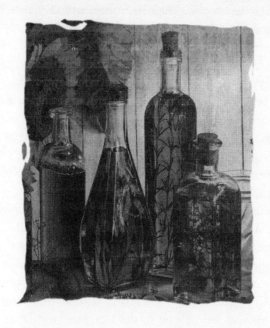

that plant products have been used since the fifteenth century
B.C. to treat cancer "should be an incentive to us in this twentieth century A.D. to search diligently into traditional medicine
and pursue the investigations with open minds."

As a matter of fact, that's precisely what scores of researchers
worldwide are doing.

In the West African nation of Ghana, pharmaceutical researchers have extracted over one dozen valuable medicines from local
plants, including the anticancer medications vincristine and vin-
blastine from the periwinkle plant; the gout remedy colchicine
from the lily; and a poison antidote called physostigmine from the
calabar bean. Although plants provide 25 percent of the medicines
in Ghana, scientists have examined fewer than 1 percent for their
medical potential. "Cultivating or sustainably harvesting these
plants could be a way to provide environmentally sound income

for people in the tropics," suggests University of Ghana botanist G.T. Odamtten, Ph.D., writing in *Medicinal Resources of the Tropical Forest* (Columbia University Press, 1996).

In the Central African country of Rwanda, where 60 to 80 percent of people consult traditional healers before heading to a physician, health officials have such respect for ethnomedical remedies that they are integrating them into health care at clinics and hospitals as well as preparing plant-based medical remedies for export. Cough syrups, medicinal teas, a disinfectant, a wound-healing ointment—they're all a part of this new push, which includes a search for plants effective against AIDS-related opportunistic infections such as tuberculosis and fungal meningitis.

Across Africa, Southeast Asia, and Latin and South America, ethnobotanists and physicians from San Francisco-based Shaman Pharmaceuticals are collecting samples of plant remedies recommended by indigenous healers, then refining the active ingredients. The company has already submitted several promising plant-derived medicines for diabetes to the U.S. Food and Drug Administration (FDA) for approval.

In a way, this long overdue investigation of African and other plants as remedies makes perfect sense. A whopping 25 percent of all prescriptions dispensed in pharmacies are for medicines containing plant-derived ingredients. For years, drug makers have taken plants with a specific healing reputation, then used the active ingredients to fashion pharmaceuticals. Numerous medicines, including aspirin (whose active ingredient is derived from the bark of willow trees) and the heart medicine digitoxin (which is derived from the dried leaves of the foxglove plant), landed on the market this way. So it shouldn't be at all surprising to find modern scientists giving thumbs-up to some of the remedies our ancestors have relied on for generations.

These researchers are telling the world what many of us already know—that traditional methods of healing can be an important resource as we seek wholeness. That's why many African Americans are looking to a variety of healing systems with new interest. Thirty years ago, you'd be hard-pressed to find many Black folks who had heard of acupuncture ("Acu-what?") or homeopathy ("It's about sex, right?"). Today we've not only discovered these and other forms of healing from different cultures, but we're redis-covering our own African healing traditions. Everywhere you look, it seems, you find Black people flocking to herb shops, asking their grandmothers about old-time remedies, or trying a prayerful healing ritual in times of need.

The Oneness of Healing Traditions

Walter H. Lewis, Ph.D., Senior Botanist at the Missouri Botanical Garden and a renowned expert on traditional plant remedies, has a favorite quote. "Someone once said that there are but two types of fools: one professes, 'This is old and therefore is good,' and the other says, 'This is new and therefore better.' Neither is necessarily correct," Lewis says. The longevity of a healing technique isn't necessarily important, or even relevant, to its value.

But you've got to admire the staying power of healing tradi-tions that have remained on the scene for hundreds, if not thou-sands, of years. If there were nothing to these traditions, surely they would have fallen by the wayside a long time ago.

If you're still cynical about traditional methods, consider for a moment how many hundreds of different cultural groups exist, or have existed at some time, on our magnificent globe. Now consider this: despite the vast differences between cultures—differences in ap-pearance, language, laws, customs, institutions, and values—there are remarkable similarities when it comes to healing traditions.

Take the concept of balance. Cultures throughout the world believe that illness represents disturbed equilibrium, where peo-ple's internal rhythms are out of tune. Once those rhythms return to harmony, health returns as well.

Let's take an example from our own culture. Black Americans who believe in ethnomedical folk remedies often speak of "high blood" or "low blood." Now, high or low blood isn't to be confused with high- or low-blood pressure. High blood refers to the volume (too much), location (too close to the head), or even the taste (too sweet) or viscosity (too thick) of a person's blood. Similarly, low blood means the blood is too scarce, too low in the body, or too bitter or thin. High blood can be caused by poor diet, especially one rich in red meat or pork. "Man cannot live by bread alone, nor pork chops neither," a Michigan minister explained to Professor Loudell Snow in *Walkin' Over Medicine* (Westview Press, 1993). "They'll run your blood up for sure." Emotional upset can cause the blood to rise, too. "When I get bogged down with worriation, I get the awfullest attack of the nerves," one Virginia homemaker explained to anthropologist Linda A. Camino, Ph.D., and colleagues. "That sends my blood up right high." It's possible to treat high blood—people use home remedies ranging from Epsom salts, garlic, and herbal teas to green vegetables, vinegar, and prayer—and prevention is a matter of avoiding the dietary or emotional excesses that cause it. In either case, the idea is to make sure that the blood avoids extremes of volume, location, taste, or consistency. People who achieve this moderation, who bring balance and stability to their blood, are blessed with good health.

Balance is the goal in India, too, where followers of Ayurvedic medicine believe that each person is a unique composite of three doshas, or body-mind types. For example, a person who suffers from chills, fever, or excessive thirst has an imbalance of pitta dosha, which influences metabolism and digestion and is associated with fire and water. Someone who's sniffling with the common cold might be said to have an overabundance of kapha dosha, which influences membranes and relates to earth and water. Based on an evaluation of a person's dosha and other considerations, Ayurvedic healers use rest, dietary restrictions, meticulously blended combinations of plant, mineral, and animal remedies, and other remedies designed to restore balance and stability.

It's a similar story in China, where people believe in the concept of *chi,* or life energy, that travels through the body in invisible channels called meridians. *Chi* normally circulates through each meridian once every twenty-four hours. Chinese healers believe we build up our supply of *chi* when we take proper care of ourselves by eating right, exercising properly, and breathing clean air. And we deplete *chi* when we're unduly influenced by life stresses—excessive cold, heat, dampness, or dryness in the environment; moods such as sorrow, anxiety, joy, or obsession; too much or too little work, exercise, or sexual activity. These stresses can block the flow of *chi* from one part of the body to another, causing an energy imbalance. The Chinese use acupuncture to unblock *chi* when it's stuck, speed it up when it's sluggish, and slow it down when it's racing. In this way, acupuncturists restore energy balance, which leads in turn to the proper functioning of every body part. (Acupressure and shiatsu work by applying pressure along the same energy meridians used in acupuncture.)

Other themes crop up again and again. Many healing traditions endorse the idea that your body knows what to do to heal itself, and that your job when you're sick is to encourage this natural healing process. Modern medicine is a notable exception: physicians often use brute force to mount an all-out assault on illness, heroically transplanting organs, engineering exquisite replacement body parts like artificial hearts and hips, and using powerful medicines whose side effects can be debilitating and sometimes even lethal. Now, doctors clearly save thousands upon thousands of lives every day, no question about it. Biomedicine has allowed the survival of countless people who, a century or even a generation ago, would have fallen victim to some deadly virus or crippling birth defect or terrible accident. So modern medicine is important in every African American's journey toward health. But many other healing traditions emphasize giving center stage to the body itself rather than to a machine or a doctor. The assumption is that we will never know more about healing than the body knows already, and that working in concert with the body's own healing rhythms is the surest ticket to wellness.

Homeopathy is a good example. A 200-year-old healing tradition originating in Germany, homeopathy is based on the Law of Similars: the same substance that in large doses produces symptoms of an illness will in very small doses cure it. Homeopathic remedies are designed to stimulate the same healing response that the body naturally generates on its own accord. Homeopathy may sound unbelievable, because it's so different from the biomedicine we've all grown up with. But whether or not you've realized it, you've probably been treated homeopathically at some point in your life: anyone who's been vaccinated against measles, influenza, or other disease has received a homeopathic remedy. Vaccines introduce a minute quantity of a virus into your body, which stimulates your immune system to produce antibodies that will protect you in case you're exposed to the real thing.

Vaccination is an accepted biomedical practice, but otherwise homeopathy and biomedicine are miles apart. With biomedical remedies, the higher the dose of a medicine, the greater the effect. In homeopathy, the more a remedy is diluted, the more potent it is. It's almost as if homeopathy says that the more gently we approach the body, the better it responds; the remedy doesn't overpower the body but it works with the body to trigger the body's natural healing response.

You can see this same respect for the body's ability to heal itself in chiropractic techniques. Chiropractors know that much of the body is under the control of the nervous system, and that the center of the nervous system is the spine, where nerves enter and exit in a pathway to the brain. The workings of the nervous system can be easily disturbed by a spinal injury, stress, illness or other problems that throw the spine out of alignment. The chiropractic goal is to bring the spine back into proper alignment, which allows the body to function normally once again.

So if you have a sprained ankle or arthritis, you can visit an orthopedic specialist. If you have mild depression or schizophrenia, you can see a psychiatrist. And if you have bursitis, menstrual difficulties, or a speech impairment, you can consult the appropriate specialists, who may indeed work wonders. But studies suggest chiropractic care can also resolve these and other health concerns. By using simple, noninvasive techniques—gentle spinal manipulation, muscle stimulation, hot packs, and ultrasound—chiropractors help the body return itself to wholeness and wellness.

There are many other examples of the universality of healing traditions. Here's one that's pretty down to earth. When we feel constipated or heavy with menstrual bloating, we're apt to reach for a laxative that flushes our bowels or a diuretic that eliminates excess fluid. Purging the body of agents that make us sick is one of the oldest and most universal healing traditions known. In North America, the Chippewa Indians fashioned enemas by steeping the inner bark of the white birch tree in hot water; the Blackfeet used the roots of the dogbane plant as a laxative. In South America, natives of what is now Guyana crushed chili peppers in water, and used that as an enema solution. In Africa, people use bamboo tubes or hollow gourds to administer similar medicines. "There is scarcely a society, primitive or otherwise, that has not used this method [enemas] as a first recourse to treatment, and to see that the concept that gave rise to it was retained in its practice we have only to consider that as recently as 200 years ago, the Christian doctrine of prayer and purging was used in cases of insanity or so-called possession," observes Christine Stockwell, author of *Nature's Pharmacy: A History of Plants and Healing* (Century, 1988). "From a modern point of view, there is little difference, other than a cultural one, between the medicine man drawing out intrusive spirits and the priest chasing out devilish influence."

These and countless other cases show that at all times and in all places, health, healing, and wholeness have been so central to human existence that all peoples have puzzled over the same basic questions: "What makes people sick?" "Why do some people prosper and flourish to a ripe age, and others die away before their time?" "How can I maintain my vitality and the well-being of my loved ones?"

These are big-picture issues, no question about it. The answers people have discovered are as diverse and colorful as the human race itself. And yet there's a certain uniformity to the principles that unite so many traditional ways of living. Whether it's a belief in the body's ability to heal itself, a careful reckoning of life's spiritual dimensions, an understanding of the need to live in balance with one's environment, or respect for the many natural remedies that surround us, the cornerstones of traditional ways are remarkably similar. Take comfort in that.

There's comfort, too, in longevity. Just as traditional African American remedies have endured the test of time, so too have the healing traditions of indigenous peoples around the world. The principles behind Whole Living stem from centuries of thoughtful deliberation by a world community. If their answers to those big-picture questions of life and healing are good enough to sustain millions of people for hundreds of years, then Whole Living can serve us well, too.

If Whole Living is our ultimate goal, what other ways of living are there? The vast majority of African Americans fall into one of three distinct lifestyles—"healthstyles" may be a better phrase. Once you learn what they are, you can begin to chart a course for your own journey to wholeness.

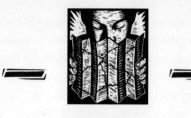

CHAPTER 2

Three Health Personalities

Now that you know more about the healing traditions that have sustained generations of African Americans and others for centuries, let's take a look at how we African Americans think about our health today. You're about to meet some fictional African Americans who typify three Health Personalities prevalent in the Black community—three very different ways of living life.

The Sickness Personality

Think of an occupation that fits the following sentence: "We'd all be a lot better off if we had fewer——."

Bet you didn't pick "doctors." Of course not. In surveys of occupational prestige, physicians consistently rank at the very top of the list. We respect doctors because they preside over the most crucial human events—birth and death, sickness and healing.

For African Americans, that respect is often tinged with uncertainty. On the one hand, we're putting our bodies and our lives on the line to a profession that's responsible for disgraces such as the Tuskegee syphilis experiment and a two-tiered "separate and unequal" medical system.

On the other hand, the brutality of slavery and the forced subservience of Jim Crow laws remain a part of our consciousness as people of color. That means we're often exceedingly respectful of authority figures and we defer to them—even when we probably shouldn't.

In the doctor's office, this ambivalence can translate into passive acceptance of whatever the doctor may say. If the physician is Dr. Perfection and never makes mistakes, we're in great shape. But if the doctor happens to schedule an unnecessary test or conduct an unwise medical procedure, we react by complaining about the physician instead of asking ourselves why we gave them the power—our power, really—to make health care decisions that affect us.

This scenario symbolizes a much larger issue, one that relates to how many African Americans approach life itself. It's an approach that has to do with issues such as how connected we feel to people around us, how committed we feel to a plan of action, and how confident we feel about getting what we need.

Here's an example. Maybe you know someone whose life seems full of frustration and despair, someone who tries hard but just can't seem to get it together. It could be your out-of-work brother-in-law, sister-girl in the work station next to yours, that brother you always see hangin' at the barber shop. Whoever it is, they look as though they're just meandering from one hard moment to the next.

Maybe the person you have in mind doesn't really understand their own abilities. Their self-esteem is tissue-thin. When you talk with them they always seem regretful about something that happened yesterday, last week, last month, or last year. And whatever their grievance may be, it always seems to be somebody else's fault.

Folks like this expect a lot from the world, and they're disappointed when they don't get it. They tend to live in the past, they focus on what they don't have, and their frustration often tempts them to seek quick fixes that rarely work. They're dependent on other people even as they blame them for making so many mistakes. They live lonely lives of frustration and despair.

These attitudes can also apply to how people think about their health. If you're the type of person who focuses on what you don't have, you might walk into a doctor's office expecting a miracle cure—then be disappointed when the heavens don't open up for you. If you depend on others but you're quick to blame them for your misfortunes, you might get overly upset when your doctor refuses to prescribe a medication you want, even though you might be depending on the medical profession for a type of healing that doctors can't really provide. If you're deeply depressed over your poor health, you might feel so despondent about your injury or illness that you can't focus on getting well: you're so stuck in the past that you can't envision a positive future.

These are all aspects of the "Sickness Personality" (see Table 1, p. 50). They're so commonplace that we often take them for granted. As a wise person once said, "Fish don't realize the water is wet"—in other words, it's hard to notice something when you're immersed in it.

TABLE 1
THREE HEALTH PERSONALITIES

Principle	Sickness Personality	Wellness Personality	Wholeness Personality
1. SELF-CONNECTEDNESS	Body focus/mind focus	Mind-body connection	Mind-body-spirit connection
2. APPROACH TO PROBLEM-SOLVING	Analysis of needs	Inventory of assets	Assumption of magnificence: all that's necessary is present
3. SOURCE OF RELIANCE	Reliance on others	Reliance on self	Reliance on God or Higher Power
4. SOURCE OF SUPPORT	Dependence	Independence	Interdependence
5. CENTEREDNESS	Not centered	Self-centered	Other-centered
6. OPTIMISM	Frequent frustration and despair	Hoping for faith	Expecting faith
7. EXPECTATIONS OF GAIN	Look to receive from others	Look to earn for self	Look to give and know you will receive
8. TIME FOCUS	Yesterday living and hope for a better day	Tomorrow living and belief that things will get better	Right now living and all you have is now!
9. SELF-REWARDS	Immediate gratification	Delayed gratification	Balance
10. COMPETITIVENESS	Competition for self-gain	Cooperation and collaboration for self-gain	Connection so that all gain
11. COMMUNITY-MINDEDNESS	"I am alone/I've got to do this myself"	"I have a network to support myself."	"We are one group."
12. PARTICIPATION IN HEALTH AND HEALING	Interest/curiosity	Involvement	Commitment
13. VITALITY LEVEL	Chronic fatigue	Energy	Enthusiasm
14. SENSE OF SELF	Self-indulgence	Self-discipline	Humility
15. SOURCE OF STRENGTH	Seek physical strength	Seek physical and psychological strength	Seek spiritual strength
16. ACCOUNTABILITY	Blame others	Take responsibility	Assume accountability

That's Joyce B.'s problem. Joyce is a young African American account executive for a prosperous advertising firm. Her career is taking off like a rocket—but her personal life looks more like a falling star. Joyce has plenty of friends and more money then she knows what to do with, but she's forever frustrated by the imperfections around her: she wants next year's raise this afternoon; she complains when her boyfriend sends her a dozen yellow roses instead of the more romantic long-stemmed reds; she moves into a new apartment and begins to groan about how she should have never left her old place. Joyce has occasional pain in her pelvis, and her gynecologist suspects it could be fibroid tumors—a diagnosis whose tentativeness Joyce finds annoying. But the doctor says that without exploratory surgery, only time will help him understand what's going on.

Now, a person who takes charge of her health might do a little research on fibroids or get a second opinion. Instead, Joyce grabs a taxi over to her favorite bistro and soothes her rumpled spirit with a double cappucino and a wedge of cheesecake, all the while moaning about having to pay such high doctors' fees for diagnoses that aren't even clearcut. She'll keep returning to that doctor, though. "He's done a lot for me over the years," she explains between bites of cheesecake. "And I don't want him to feel that I'm being disloyal by questioning him."

Joyce shows at least five signs of the Sickness Personality. She relies completely on her doctor (Principle #3: Source of reliance) and depends on others to solve her problems (Principle #4: Source of support). She looks to receive from other people (Principle #7: Expectations of gain), she expects immediate gratification from her physician despite hazy medical circumstances (Principle #9: Self-rewards), and she's only mildly interested in resolving her own health concerns (Principle #12: Participation in health and healing).

None of this should come as any great surprise: many of us are like Joyce B. African Americans have been denied decent health care for so long that when we finally do get a good doctor, it's easy to feel unnecessarily grateful, fiercely loyal, and full of expectation for a quick fix. That sense of gratitude and loyalty may be one reason that we can be slow to assert our health needs.

The Sickness Personality may be widespread, but the assumptions it's based on are flawed. See if you agree:

Assumption 1: People with a Sickness Personality look for immediate gratification. They stroll into a doctor's office like they're pulling up to the window at a fast-food restaurant. It's as though they want a little packet of "instant health crystals" that they can tear open and sprinkle into a glass of juice.

Flaw: If only genuine health were so automatic. Think about it: if getting healthy were as easy as ordering a bag of french fries, wouldn't everyone you know be healthy?

Assumption 2: People with a Sickness Personality depend on health professionals. After all, they're the experts, right? They're the ones who go to school for umpteen years to earn the credentials that signify they're qualified to make us healthy.

Flaw: If you rely on someone else to make you healthy, your health is limited by the skill of your doctor—a human being who is not, after all, God. Besides, if you place all of your healing power in the hands of someone else, don't you think it's easy to lose sight of what you can do to advance your own health?

Assumption 3: People with a Sickness Personality look to receive. Their health depends on others giving them something, whether that "something" is helpful medical advice, good genes, respectful treatment in the doctor's office, or whatever.

Flaw: Sure, it's reasonable to expect sound medical advice and healthy respect from the people who are paid to give it. But life—and health—are more than about getting good service—or *getting* in general. Otherwise, you'd never find a perfectly healthy African American elder who's never been to a doctor. Our wiser elders understand that there's a lot we can do as individuals to ensure our well-being. One of them is giving to others. After all, if everyone were out for number one, we might as well shut down the Black community and lock the door behind us, because our existence as a people has always depended on being there for each other.

Assumption 4: People with a Sickness Personality see the body as isolated parts. Doctors become specialists so they can learn a lot about people's hearts, their kidneys, or some other body part. We follow their lead by thinking about one part of our bodies as separate from other parts. It's a lot simpler that way.

Flaw: It may be simple, but it's also simplistic. People aren't automobiles; we're more than an assemblage of parts. We're made of complex interconnected systems, many of them irreplaceable. That's why you need an M.D. degree before you can be a psychiatrist—you can't understand what's going on in someone's mind without appreciating what's happening throughout their body.

Assumption 5: People with a Sickness Personality go it alone. They navigate the health care system alone, they plead with their insurance company to cover second opinions alone, they alone are responsible for getting themselves to the doctor for checkups.

Flaw: Carrying full responsibility for anything—and certainly something as important as our health—all by ourselves can be a pretty lonely affair. After all, humans are social animals. Rarely do you find a happy hermit. Most of us are truly content only when we're with people who love us and who'll prevent us from being lonely, especially in our hour of need: when we're ill.

The point is that we live in a culture where the expectations people place on themselves and others may be unrealistic. People with a Sickness Personality may not realize it, but there's no such thing as a quick fix. It's unreasonable to expect others to care more about us than we do ourselves. Living in the past can be a way of avoiding the future. Looking for a handout makes us forget our own power. Blaming others can mean we're avoiding taking responsibility ourselves. Assuming we're alone in the world does nothing but isolate us from those who care about us.

The problem with the Sickness Personality is that it's . . . well, it's about sickness—being sick, staying sick, feeling sick of being sick, blaming the world for making us sick, relying on other people to stop us from feeling sick. There's not too much that's healthy about it. That's why when it comes to thinking about our health more and more African Americans are turning to alternatives.

The Wellness Personality

What kinds of alternatives are we talking about? Well, breaking out of the Sickness Personality can mean different things to different people. But more and more African Americans are seeking answers in so-called alternative medicine. They realize that while biomedicine is well suited for certain health problems, alternatives to biomedicine are better suited for others. These alternatives— many of them traditional healing approaches used for centuries— are numerous and diverse. Some alternative treatments—such as acupuncture, homeopathy, massage, and reflexology—work on the body's energy fields. Others—such as herbal therapy and vitamin and nutrition therapy—provide a proper balance of nutrients, hormones, and enzymes that help the body operate efficiently. Still others—such as biofeedback, prayer, and meditation—integrate the mental and spiritual side of healing. The alternatives you'll soon read about in Part Two ("Ways to Heal") work with the body's own natural rhythms instead of trying to control those rhythms with harsh medicines and toxic therapies. They respect the body's ability to heal itself rather than try to impose a healing regimen on it. They also take into account the wonderful, complete, whole person that you are, instead of focusing on just one or two body parts.

Let's call this health personality, the one that brings alternative therapies into the picture, the "Wellness Personality."

Now, the Wellness Personality has a lot going for it, especially when you compare it with the Sickness Personality. Where Sickness views the body and mind as separate, Wellness brings them together. For example, aromatherapists will tell you that inhaling oil extracted from a rose or an orange has a tranquilizing effect on the body. At the other end of the spectrum, oils drawn from basil, rosemary, and several other spice plants stimulate the body. How can a mere aroma have such an effect on your entire system? Well, aromatherapy capitalizes on the ability of the essential oils from plants to trigger certain brain signals that in turn affect the workings of bodily processes. In aromatherapy, as in so many alternative approaches, the mind and body are one integrated unit.

Here's another advantage. Whereas the Sickness Personality stands for immediate gratification and self-indulgence (remember Joyce B.'s cheesecake?), the Wellness Personality represents delayed gratification and self-discipline. That comes in pretty handy when the health goal you're striving for cannot arrive overnight. For instance, it may take several sessions or longer, depending on the health challenge you're facing, to achieve results from an acupuncturist, chiropractor, or other alternative practitioner. Alternative treatments are generally gentler than biomedicine, plus your body can take a while to respond to them if you're accustomed to fast-acting biomedicine. So alternative approaches take a little patience and self-discipline, but the benefits are often well worth it.

And a third advantage: Wellness replaces the loneliness of sickness with networks of kindred spirits. Someone at the beauty shop or at the gym may stop you and mention a herbal remedy because they know you're bothered by headaches or anxiety or premenstrual syndrome. The next thing you know, you're comparing notes with a circle of mutual friends who are all interested in herbal therapies. You trade information on where to buy high-quality herbs at a reasonable price; you chat about good herbal reference books; and when you begin to grow your own herbs, folks encourage you along. By adopting the Wellness Personality, you've replaced the loneliness of the Sickness Personality with camaraderie and warmth.

The Wellness Personality changes how we think about competition, too. The dog-eat-dog mentality of modern life encourages us to think of others not as human beings, but as competitors for the same resources that we want for ourselves, whether that means money, a good job, decent housing, a college education, or a fine mate. In fact, our lives are filled with competition that symbolizes self-gain at the expense of others. No wonder so many of us burn out with ulcers, viral illnesses, and other stress-induced illnesses! In contrast, the Wellness Approach encourages something entirely different: cooperation and collaboration as a way to achieve what we need.

You can see how Wellness really is light-years ahead of the old Sickness model. Think of it. Once you're armed with alternative routes to health, you can begin to replace dependence on the health care system with newfound independence—combining reliance on others with reliance on yourself. That way, you can take responsibility instead of blaming others, you have a reason to look to tomorrow instead of being stuck in the past, and you can focus on your assets instead of your needs.

Likewise, once you accept the body-mind connection, you stop looking for physical strength alone, and turn your sights instead to achieving physical and psychological strength. You begin to renew your body and your mind, bringing vitality to both. Once you do that, a life of malaise or boredom or chronic fatigue can become charged with energy, as interest in merely repairing your health turns to involvement in maintaining it.

Now, this may surprise you—but as good as it is, Wellness

has a few kinks. What could be wrong with an approach that delivers such a terrific payoff?

For one thing, people with Wellness Personalities can lack balance. Say hello to Harriet P., an insurance company secretary. After several false starts, Harriet decided that she was going to do something once and for all about her weight. No more would she sacrifice her health by loading up on diet pills, she promised. No longer would she try in vain to soothe her disappointment over her size by (ironically) plunging into a platter of fried chicken wings or downing a quart of mint chocolate chip ice cream. She resolved to eat less red meat and fewer sugary, greasy indulgences, and to make friends with fruits and vegetables, beans, and whole grains. She also started going out for walks with several overweight friends who got together five mornings a week at a local high-school track. Harriet was serious about these important changes in her life—and it showed: in just ten months, she lost nearly sixty pounds.

Harriet was looking good and feeling strong—until a phone conversation one day with her sister, Sheila, who's two years her junior. The two were reminiscing laughingly about Sheila's eighth birthday party—the one when the cake Harriet had inexpertly baked for her emerged from the oven looking like Elvis's pompadour. Harriet suddenly felt uncomfortable and abruptly steered the conversation in another direction. That's when she first realized how vigorously she avoided talking about that phase of her childhood. Soon after the birthday party, Harriet's uncle had begun to sexually abuse her. The abuse lasted for more than a year. "Those were terrifying months for me," she recalls. "It took me a long time to realize that a lot of my adult behavior—like my compulsive eating, which was a sign of craving control and comfort—were tied to those early experiences."

Harriet had made important strides toward Wellness even before the phone conversation with her sister. She had replaced the immediate gratification and self-indulgence of comfort foods with the delayed gratification and self-discipline of a long-term eating and exercise plan. She had moved from feeling isolated by her weight to being connected with others who shared a similar commitment to change. That helped her break her fixation on how miserable she'd been about her size, and gave her a reason to think hopefully about tomorrow.

But while Harriet's commitment to good nutrition and exercise had given her physical and emotional health an unmistakable boost, she had neglected her spiritual side. And it was her spirit, her most precious inner self, that had taken the brunt of the sexual assaults. Over time—and with the help of an excellent psychotherapist—Harriet realized that it was futile to try to manage her weight without addressing the underlying abuse that contributed to her eating patterns. Only a commitment to all three parts of her—the physical, the mental, and the spiritual—would bring her the genuine healing she craved. "My therapist told me, 'A man who's in perfect physical health can still go home and beat his wife,'" recalls Harriet. "That tells me how important it is to cultivate a good spirit."

The second problem with the Wellness Personality, and one that relates to the lack of balance, is that Wellness isn't necessarily comprehensive. Take a look at Ron M., a twenty-seven-year-old plumber. One day, Ron's fishing buddy Clarence starts to rave about how vitamins have helped him tackle a persistent skin problem. Ron figures vitamins might help clear up his own skin, which has been oily and embarrassingly pimple-prone since adolescence. So he checks out a book on natural remedies from his public library and heads to a local natural foods store for a fistful of vitamin supplements.

A week goes by, and no change. Three weeks, and nothing. Two whole months elapse. Not a thing. Every morning when Ron looks in the mirror, the same oily face looks back at him.

Ron mentions his frustration the next time he and his friend are out at the lake. Clarence asks, "Are you still doing that same double-bacon-cheeseburger-and-fries thing you used to do before you took the vitamins?"

"Now, you know that's my favorite lunch," admits Ron.

"And what about your exercise routine?" Clarence asks. "Do you have one yet?"

"Not yet, but hey—what does that have to do with my skin?"

"Answer me this," replies Clarence, "Have you ever closed your eyes and just imagined what your skin would look like if it were healthy?"

"Man, what you talkin' about?" asks Ron, incredulous. "Only time I close my eyes is when I fall asleep."

Ron expects a few vitamins to compensate for what could be three major contributors to his problem skin: a greasy diet, a sedentary lifestyle, and a lack of spiritual involvement in his healing. He assumes he'll get the results he wants by changing one element in his life (and a pretty easy element at that) instead of taking a hard look at the big picture, and making a more substantial investment in his health. And that's a second limitation of the Wellness Personality. Wellness doesn't necessarily commit all of your energy to achieving health, because it doesn't draw on every resource. Wellness can mean getting a massage once a week or experimenting with a homeopathic remedy during cold and flu season—but doing little else to change how you think about your health. In other words, as good as Wellness is, it can represent a less-than-total commitment to health and healing.

Ron's attitude is actually pretty common. Having grown up in a fast-food environment, a culture where everything from bank transactions to wedding ceremonies are often reduced to their stripped-down essentials in the name of efficiency, we often think of visiting even a chiropractor or herbalist or homeopath with the same "heal me" expectations that we often have when we visit a physician. Just like in the Sickness Personality, this approach removes the responsibility for our health from our own hands and places it in someone else's. To take full advantage of the opportunities of alternative healing, we need to move from involvement to commitment, from approaching health with mere energy to approaching it with full-fledged enthusiasm.

Let's move beyond Wellness to an exciting approach that can help you find optimal health and healing, an approach that helps you realize your whole potential. We'll call it the Wholeness Personality.

The Wholeness Personality

To picture Wholeness in action, imagine the life of a sixty-two-year-old grandmother we'll call Patricia B. Patricia lives in a housing project in a crumbling section of what was at one time a fairly vigorous inner city. She has a touch of arthritis here and there, and she's had diabetes for most of her adult life.

At one time Patricia used to be an assembly-line worker making $15.50 an hour at a nearby manufacturing plant. But a few years ago the company relocated nearly 2,000 jobs to Mexico and Nicaragua to cut labor costs. Since then, Patricia, who had just finished high school when her first child was born and never had the chance to attend college, has been unable to find full-time work. She makes do by piecing together three part-time jobs—a makeshift arrangement that brings eight- to twelve-hour days, lengthy cross-town bus commutes, minimal job security, and no health insurance.

As Langston Hughes would say, Patricia's life ain't no crystal stair. But you wouldn't know it by looking at her. A tall, mahogany-skinned woman who describes herself as "built for comfort, not for speed," Patricia holds her head high as she climbs the stairs to her third-floor apartment. The elevator has been out for the past year, she explains. But she sees the disrepair as an opportunity. "I don't mind the exercise," she says with a smile.

Patricia's daughter is serving time for a narcotics violation, and Patricia hasn't seen the children's father in years. Until her daughter gets her life together, Patricia is mother and grandmother to two preschoolers, ages 2 and 3. Ever since she assumed her new role, Patricia has found a way to make sure the kids get their immunizations and doctor's checkups on time, even if it means spending half of a Saturday riding buses to get to the clinic. "We take coloring books and little sandwiches and call it a picnic," she explains.

When the kids come down with an ailment that Patricia senses a doctor won't know much about, she consults Miss Lydia, an elderly herbalist and spiritualist who lives a couple of blocks away. "Lydia knows there's a lot more to being healthy than what they teach them youngsters in medical school," Patricia says, settling into a vinyl-covered easy chair in her small but tidy living room. She tells of a time when the children were hit almost simultaneously by a mysterious sickness that left them restless and unable to eat or drink. Miss Lydia listened to the symptoms, then went out into her little yard where she grows a few herbs. "Steep this in some hot water and have dem chirren drink it every night for three nights," she said, handing Patricia some leaves. The herbs seemed to comfort the kids and soothe their stomachs. Within two days their appetite was back.

Shaniqua, Patricia's best friend and next-door neighbor, admires this grandparent who's so full of life. "Patricia is just really confident and comfortable in the world—even though life isn't easy for her, you know what I'm saying," she explains. "She lets her spirit guide her in all things, whether it's planning a nutritious menu on a budget, or caring for a group of neighborhood kids three nights a week so their mothers can take G.E.D. classes."

Patricia's life may not be comfortable, either financially or emotionally. Like every African American, she has worries and concerns, and she knows it would surely be nice to have more help. But life for Patricia contains all of the elements of wholeness.

For instance, Patricia has never thought of her body as being separate from her mind (the Sickness Personality) and she figured out long ago that the mind-body connection (the Wellness Personality) leaves out a key ingredient: the spirit. So when things get tough—life is life, after all—she prays not just for physical strength (the Sickness Personality) or physical and psychological strength (the Wellness Personality), but for strength on all three planes—physical, psychological, and spiritual. This belief and trust in the spirit lets Patricia move beyond relying on others (the Sickness Personality), and beyond self-reliance (the Wellness Personality). Instead, she places faith in her Creator, trusting that a force much larger than her will help her provide (the Wholeness Personality).

Likewise, Patricia doesn't spend time taking an inventory of what she needs, and bemoaning the fact that she doesn't have it (the Sickness Personality). And unlike some upwardly mobile Black folks, she doesn't obsess over what she has (Wellness Personality). Instead, despite her financial poverty, she assumes a magnificence of riches, and that she already has everything she needs to live a full and gratifying existence (Wholeness Personality).

For example, her diabetic relatives—she has three of them—frequently complain about how difficult it is to manage the illness. They feel that interrupting their lives for the seemingly constant injections of insulin is nothing but a bother—and an expensive one at that. Patricia, on the other hand, understands that managing her diabetes is not about the money she may not have; she knows that what she needs is already in her hands. Or more precisely, in her feet—which she uses to walk five city blocks to and from the corner grocery store instead of catching the bus to the store. She's followed this routine ever since her doctor told her that people with diabetes who eat intelligently and who exercise their way to a lower weight often see such a drastic improvement in their body's use of insulin that they no longer need to rely on store-bought injections. That's how Patricia moves beyond her relatives, who seem to talk forever about what they need (the Sickness Personality). She doesn't bother taking inventory of what she has (the Wellness Personality), because she knows that whatever she needs is already hers (the Wholeness Personality).

Some folks who used to work the assembly line with Patricia grumble about how much easier things were in the good old days, when jobs were plentiful and pay was generous. But not Patricia. She doesn't dwell on the past (the Sickness Personality). And she doesn't live for tomorrow, investing everything in her hopes (the Wellness Personality). Patricia lives in the moment, knowing that right now is all she has, trusting that each and every day is what she makes it. This way, she doesn't blame others when things don't go according to plan (the Sickness Personality). And she avoids merely taking responsibility for how events unfold (the Wellness Personality). Instead, she feels fully accountable for how she makes her way through the day's events (the Wholeness Personality).

Instead of feeling locked in head-to-head competition with her neighbors—for a full-time job, for example—(the Sickness Personality), or simply collaborating with others for self-gain (the Wellness Personality), Patricia connects with people around her so that everyone gains. It's easy for her to babysit her neighbors' kids, she figures, because when one of us wins, we all win. This way, Patricia doesn't feel the loneliness of the Sickness Personality, and she gains much more than just the supportive network that she would get under the Wellness Personality. No, her reward is much higher: She feels at one with her community, her family, herself, and her God. That's why instead of merely looking to receive (the Sickness Personality) or looking to earn (the Wellness Personality), Patricia looks to give (the Wholeness Personality). It's by giving that she knows she will receive.

Patricia also incorporates more than one healing approach into her life. She uses a biomedical healer for some health problems and an ethnomedical healer for others. Unlike Ron the plumber, she knows better than to rely on a single healing method. Life is more complex than that. She also understands that a truly healthy approach to life takes a total commitment. So she eats thoughtfully—she calls herself a semivegetarian and she really watches her fat intake; she makes it a point to fit as much exercise as she can into her busy day; and from time to time she finds comfort at the end of her day by "talking" with her Aunt Ellie, a favorite relative who provided Patricia with a listening ear and endless wisdom while she was alive.

Notice how many elements of Patricia's life aren't that different from the traditional African ways explained in Chapter 1. Like her African ancestors, Patricia places faith in the interconnectedness of community. She realizes that the spirits of her loved ones remain with her, and she feels just as connected to them as she did when they were living. She believes in the interweaving of mind, body and spirit, and in the nonjudgmental flexibility it takes to pursue whatever remedies that do the trick, whether they be ethnomedical or biomedical.

In fact, you might say that despite formidable obstacles, Patricia fully understands what it takes to live a full, vibrant, peaceful, happy life. Patricia—and many African Americans like her—approach health and healing in the fullest, most complete sense of the words. They're the ones who understand the real meaning of holistic health.

What is Holistic Health?

You've probably heard that term before. Holistic health is a catch-all phrase with multiple meanings. Holistic health might be synonymous with eating organic foods, or setting aside time each day to meditate. It may mean bringing a spiritual focus to your life, or seeking out alternative healers like chiropractors and massage therapists.

One way to appreciate the meaning of holistic health is to think for a moment about what the word "health" means to you. Lots of people consider themselves healthy if they don't have an illness or disease. Under this definition, anyone who doesn't have the flu, high blood pressure, cancer, or any other problem you could find in a medical textbook qualifies as being healthy. That's one definition.

Many African Americans think about health a little differently. We're apt to say we're healthy as long as we can make it through the day doing what we need to do. As long as we can function well enough to make it to work, take care of the kids, get to church, and pay the bills, that's good enough for us. So when a doctor tells us we have hypertension, or says we need regular checkups for cancer, we may wonder what the fuss is all about. "I don't feel sick," we might say to ourselves.

Well, health in a holistic sense does mean the absence of disease. It also means the ability to function. But it means so much more. Take a deep breath and relax your mind for a moment. Now close your eyes and think back to a time in your life when you felt most alive, a time when you felt boundless energy or great surges of creativity. Imagine your body feeling flexible and powerful, capable of magnificent daily miracles, great and small. Picture yourself having the curiosity of a child, the vitality of a teenager, and the understanding of the wisest elder. Think of how comforting and reassuring it feels knowing that your every step on earth is guided by a watchful hand that ensures that your every need is met.

If you're like most people, you may be smiling right now. And rightly so: what you are visualizing is supremely pleasant. That image of happy, powerful confidence and vitality that you've conjured in your mind is the ultimate goal of holistic health.

(Notice how much richer and fuller this goal is than simply being disease-free or simply being able to function.) Living your life holistically means achieving balance, fullness, interconnections, inner hope, inner strength, and inner peace.

How do you reach that goal? That's where the Wholeness Personality comes in. Holistic health means moving beyond Sickness, through Wellness, into Wholeness. When you live according to the Wholeness principles outlined in this chapter, you'll find yourself living to the fullest. And that's what it means to have Whole Living.

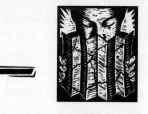

CHAPTER 3

Whole Living—Getting It, Doing it, Loving It

Every journey brings two questions: "Where am I going?" and "How do I get there?" When you're reorienting your health—reorienting your life, really—the first question is pretty easy: Where am I going? "I want to Live Wholly."

It's the second question that's a head-scratcher: So how do I get there from here? Let's take a look at one person's journey to see how he did it. We'll call him Calvin T.

Calvin was a popular and outgoing college senior, an athletic, energetic young brother whose childhood dream of becoming an architect seemed on the verge of bearing fruit until one night in early April. It was the end of "Freaknique," the spring break hangout in Atlanta, Georgia, for hordes of African American college students. Calvin was cruising through an intersection when his car was struck from the side by a reckless driver who claimed he didn't see the light.

At first, Calvin felt relieved that the only casualty seemed to be his car door, which crumpled like aluminum foil. But later that night he realized something was very wrong with his back. The pain started with a small ache but by the next morning, recalls the husky soft-spoken young man, "My back felt like it was on fire."

The doctors did a CAT scan and found that one of Calvin's spinal disks was bulging and probably pressing on a nerve. That might explain the pain, they said, though it was hard to be sure; many people have bulging disks that never cause them any trouble, and Calvin's could have been like this for years. At first, the physicians suggested rest, painkillers as needed, and mild exercise to prevent his back muscles from weakening and making the problem worse. That seemed to quiet the pain for a while, but getting rid of it was a different story. After weeks of trying this therapy and that, the best the doctors seemed able to do was to offer injections of nerve-deadening medicine, which helped only temporarily but soon wore off.

Calvin managed to graduate on time, but in the months that followed he slipped into a depression. The near-constant pain was bad enough, but the pain was also a bitter reminder that one night of partying in Atlanta may have been the last carefree moment he was ever destined to have. "I was a 21-year-old college grad with good grades and everything to look forward to, and suddenly I'm flat on my back," Calvin remembers. "I felt like I had been cheated out of my future." Calvin vented his resentment on his doctors and even his family, blaming them for not doing enough to help him, for not caring. He couldn't stop thinking about the years before his accident, when his life was so much simpler and easier, when his face usually registered an easy smile rather than frequent winces.

In desperation, Calvin turned inward, medicating his hurt with marijuana. Charlie, one of Calvin's favorite uncles, had cancer at the time, and his doctor had prescribed marijuana to fight the nausea of chemotherapy. "I thought, hey, if it's good enough for

Uncle Charlie, it's good enough for me," Calvin recalls. "I mean, I had something pretty powerful eating away at me, too."

Ironically, it was Charlie who snapped Calvin out of it. "I was visiting him in the intensive care unit—he was pretty sick at the time—and he turned to me and said, 'I can see how much pain you're in,'" Calvin remembers. "I mean, here was a man who was dying of cancer, and all I could think about was my aching back."

The incident was an epiphany of sorts for Calvin. It helped him appreciate how fortunate he was to be living and breathing on this earth, and it inspired him to take inventory of the positives in his life. Calvin resolved to try to take more responsibility for managing his health. He found a support group for chronic pain sufferers where he met new friends who helped him understand that life goes on despite mishaps like his. In fact, he realized by listening to others' stories that life goes on despite utter disasters, like near-fatal accidents and life-threatening diseases. Months of despair began turning to hope. He learned to be patient with his body and to listen more to its needs instead of being driven by his own wants. In the old days, despite his accident, he wouldn't think twice about heading down to the beach to water-ski with his friends—only to pay for it with a week of fresh spasms of pain. "Nowadays if I choose to join my friends, I take along my new hobby—a camera—and snap pictures of them having near-death experiences," says Calvin with a smile.

On the advice of a former college roommate, a young fellow from Taiwan, Calvin looked into acupuncture. After a month or so of twice-weekly visits to an acupuncturist, Calvin realized that the needle technique was for real. He couldn't believe how effectively a few minutes of treatment blocked his pain. "Acupuncture made a believer out of me," Calvin says. "Compared to the injections I had been getting from my physician, the acupuncture appointments were briefer, the treatment was less expensive, and the relief lasted a lot longer."

Calvin's happy experience with acupuncture opened the door to experimenting with other alternative therapies. Some worked better than others; reflexology and deep-tissue massage seemed to benefit his back the most. For the first time in months, he found himself actually looking forward to the future.

As he continued to explore new routes to health, Calvin also discovered the joy of giving back. It happened one summer afternoon when his landlady, Miss Effie, a kindly retired schoolteacher who's as fond of Calvin as she is of her own children, brought him a handful of fresh-cut daisies from her garden. It was her way of thanking him for recommending that she visit an acupuncturist for her aching arthritic hip. "Miss Effie was so grateful. She said she felt half her age!" Calvin recalls. "That's when I realized how wonderful it can be to make a meaningful contribution to other people's lives."

Nearly two years after the accident, Calvin is a different guy. He's not entirely free of pain, but several things have helped him come to peace with it; he considers that genuine health. For instance, he's a much more spiritual fellow these days. A book on Zen Buddhism has helped him live in the present, and to accept whatever life brings him at any given moment, whether that moment means pain or relief. He's also learning to distinguish between the health concerns that his physician can address and those that an alternative practitioner is better suited for. Finally, by giving to others—by volunteering on Saturday afternoons at a local pain-treatment clinic, for example—he's begun to feel more connected with the community around him. "It's ironic," Calvin says. "Even though I still feel physical discomfort from time to time, I think of myself as being healthier than before the accident."

Getting to Wholeness

Calvin didn't deliberately set out to travel from Sickness to Wellness to Wholeness, but that's what he ended up doing. He moved from despair over his accident to hope about coping with it; from looking to receive to looking to give; from being dependent on others to recognizing the interdependence of those around him. During that evolution, Calvin learned to live for the moment instead of in the past, and to be accountable for his health instead of blaming others.

Lots of African Americans are discovering exciting new dimensions of health through Whole Living. Just as no two people and no two circumstances are alike, no two paths to wholeness are identical. But for most folks, the journey to Wholeness involves similar stepping stones. You can launch your own personal program to live fully, healthily, and wholly in just five easy steps:

Step #1:   Identify your health personality.

Step #2:   Ask yourself how effectively modern medicine (biomedicine) is addressing your health concerns.

Step #3:   Identify the health concerns that may be good candidates for alternative healing approaches.

Step #4:   Read the entries in Part Three that apply to your health concerns.

Step #5:   Plan a strategy using your Health Personality score.

It's simple! All you need is paper and pencil, an hour or two of uninterrupted time, and your imagination to envision your new health possibilities.

Let's walk through the process step by step.

Step #1:   Identify Your Health Personality

If you're lost on the freeway, that badly folded road map from your glove compartment won't be much good until you can figure out where on the map you happen to be. The same goes for your health. Unless you understand where you are, you won't be able to get to where you're going.

Of course, it's not always easy to recognize where we stand. That's where the Health Personality Quiz comes in (p. 7). It's designed to show your present location on the Sickness-Wellness-Wholeness spectrum. If you haven't already taken the quiz, spend a few moments and do so now.

The quiz questions refer to the principles that appear in Table 1 (p. 50). Here's how to score the quiz and interpret your answers:

To Score

For every odd-numbered question, give yourself:

    1 point for each (a) answer,

    2 points for each (b) answer,

    3 points for each (c) answer.

For every even-numbered question, give yourself:

    3 points for each (a) answer,

    2 points for each (b) answer,

    1 point for each (c) answer.

The total is your Health Personality Score. If your total score is:

51–60 You have a Wholeness Personality and are Whole Living. Congratulations!

45–50 You're in transition between Wellness and Wholeness. Your goal is very close!

36–44 You have a Wellness Personality. With a little more effort, you can be Whole Living!

30–35 You're between Sickness and Wellness. You're moving in the right direction!

20–29 You have a Sickness Personality. But don't despair! Once you move toward Wellness and Wholeness, you'll be amazed at how much better you can feel!

Step #2: Ask Yourself How Effectively Modern Medicine (Biomedicine) Is Addressing Your Health Concerns

Most of us are born into the biomedical system—literally. A physician brings us into this world, and from that moment on we think of doctors as indispensable members of our community. And they are. Physicians are excellently suited to handle certain medical conditions, especially health emergencies such as broken bones, gunshot wounds, diabetic comas, heart attacks, and stroke. African American physicians in particular have a stellar record of providing compassionate care in ways that are sensitive to what their Black patients are going through.

But as we've noted before, no healing system is perfect; biomedicine is no exception. For example, modern medicine isn't particularly effective at handling chronic disease. Biomedicine does offer life-saving medicines that help to control such long-term health problems as high blood pressure and glaucoma. But if doctors were as effective at preventing chronic illnesses as they are at performing crisis medicine, we wouldn't lose hundreds of thousands of African Americans prematurely each year to heart disease, cancer, hypertension, kidney failure, and other gradual killers.

Biomedicine has other weaknesses. For one, it compartmentalizes the body. Physicians are trained to see bodies as individual parts rather than interconnected wholes, even though the heart that a cardiologist listens to, the ankle that an orthopedic surgeon feels, or the nerves that a neurologist tests are connected to a living, breathing, whole person. Which is why it often makes sense to find a healing method that respects the whole person, a method such as acupuncture, nutrition therapy, or the other alternative approaches outlined in Part Two.

Modern medicine often doesn't take into account our individuality, either. If the truth be known, patients are as unique as their fingerprints. Take cigarette smokers, for instance. Studies show that people who smoke are less likely to get lung cancer if they have a diet that's rich in vitamin A or if they're emotionally well grounded, compared to smokers with lousy diets or poor emotional health. Likewise, the nutritional needs within a given group of twenty or so people can vary by as much as 700 percent depending on a person's age, activity level, stress level, and similar factors, according to the late Roger Williams, Ph.D., author of *Biochemical Individuality* (University of Texas Press, 1980). Despite this wide variability, doctors typically use a "cookie-cutter" approach to treating patients. "The conventional doctor who has twelve patients with asthma will often provide each of them with the same recommendations and prescription drugs, in effect treating the condition and not the patients themselves," explains Leon Chaitow, N.D., D.O., of London, England, in *Alternative Medicine; The Definitive Guide* (Future Medicine, 1995).

The danger of the cookie-cutter approach becomes clear when you consider that asthma can have many potential causes. If the wheezing and airway tightening is caused by an allergic reaction to dust or pet hair, why ask patients to pay for expensive inhalation treatment when what they really need is a good housecleaning? If stress and anxiety bring on asthma attacks, why use prescription medicines to force open the airways when you could go to the source with stress-relieving massage therapy? If the problem is a misaligned spine that's pressing on the nerves that serve the lungs, why focus on the lungs when what the patient really needs is chiropractic treatments to realign the spine and relieve pressure on the nerves?

You can see how the alternative healing approaches outlined in Part Two fill a void by giving us routes to healing and wholeness that biomedicine simply doesn't provide. If you have a Wellness Personality or Wholeness Personality, chances are you've already figured this out.

But no matter what your health personality may be, you can come closer to Whole Living by distinguishing between the things biomedicine does well for you and the things it doesn't. Spend a few moments right now to assess your relationship with the biomedical system. Take a mental inventory of your health concerns—and think of the word "health" in its broadest possible sense to cover emotional and spiritual well-being as well as physical well-being.

For example, if Calvin T.—that young student—were doing this exercise, he might list as his health concerns "chronic back pain," "depression," and "feeling isolated and disappointed." If Patricia B.—the grandmother and former assembly-line worker—were doing it, she might write, "arthritis," "diabetes," and "worry over security of my grandchildren." Jot down these concerns in a column along the left side of a sheet of paper.

Now ask yourself how helpful modern medicine has been in addressing these concerns. Use a 1 to 5 scale, with 1 meaning "not very helpful" and 5 signifying "extremely helpful." Be sure to record the reason(s) for each score. You don't have to write down your health concerns in any particular order; just record them as they come to mind. If you aren't using biomedicine to address a certain health concern, give that entry a 0.

Here's a sample list from Glenda F., a thirty-two-year-old high-school librarian and single mother of two children, one of whom (Malcolm) has sickle-cell disease and has been classified by his second-grade teacher as having a learning disability. Glenda has moderate hypertension, a family history of cancer, and is outgoing and friendly although she wrestles with depression. She is 5'4" and weighs 210 pounds. She scored a 31 on the Health Personality Quiz, indicating she's in transition between Sickness and Wellness.

Glenda F.:

My health concerns: How helpful is biomedicine?

My weight: 1—My doctor always tells me to lose weight, but he always seems too busy to explain how. Plus, I don't think he understand how hard it is for me to change my eating habits.

Malcolm's sickle cell anemia: 5—Working with the pediatrician has been great. Sometimes when Malcolm has episodes of pain, we have to visit the emergency room, but the staff knows their stuff.

Depression/my spirit: 2—Antidepressant medicines make me too "crazy" (agitated), feels too heavy so I don't like to take them.

Hypertension: 2—My medicine (diuretic) is effective but causes lots of bathroom trips!

Too much "worriation":   1—Too bad there's no medicine that will help pay bills, etc. Also, I worry about Malcolm. Does he really have a learning disability, or is his White teacher too quick to judge Black kids?

Occasional stomachache: 4—Antacids work OK.

Cancer: 4—I get Pap smears and I don't smoke. But I wish I could do more to prevent cancer.

Step #3:   Identify the Health Concerns That May Be Good Candidates for Alternative Healing Approaches
Once you've recorded your health concerns and assigned each one a score, mark the concerns that have scores lower than 5. Now turn to the table of contents of this book and discover the many alternative healing approaches in Part Two that you can use to address them.

For Glenda, biomedicine rates a 5 ("extremely helpful") for Malcolm's sickle cell anemia. But all of her other health concerns earn ratings less than 5. So she turns to the table of contents and moves down the remainder of her list. Alternative approaches might be good for these concerns.

Step #4: *Read the Entries in Part Three That Apply to Your Health Concerns*

Part Three contains easy-to-understand information about dozens of health concerns that can be addressed using alternative healing techniques. Read through the sections that are relevant to your concerns. When Glenda pages through Part Three, she finds many alternative healing options for depression, hypertension, and cancer; her weight falls under "obesity," and "worriation" comes under stress. If you're interested in learning more about a particular healing technique (such as acupuncture, reflexology, etc.), you'll find a description in Part Two.

For any given health concern on your list, you may discover that Part Three provides more information than you need. Not to worry. You don't have to digest it all; just try to come away with a feel for the options that are available to you.

Try to get a sense, too, of which options sound the most appealing. For example, Glenda has many ways she can handle her high blood pressure. Under nutrition therapy, she can boost her intake of potassium and magnesium while cutting down on her sodium. That really floats her boat, because she adores sweet potatoes, greens, bananas, melons, and other luscious fruits and vegetables. She feels good about seeking out an African American herb doctor, too. Their knowledge of additional plant-based cures— garlic, for example—may help. On the other hand, although aromatherapy offers some interesting remedies for hypertension, she'd feel more comfortable using essential oils for the immediate relief of short-term health problems. "This way, I won't be telling myself a thousand times a day, 'Shouldn't you be using your aromatherapy oils?' " Glenda says. "I'd drive myself stone crazy."

Finally, bear in mind which alternative practitioners are available to you. While many alternative therapies are completely suitable for self-care, others—like acupuncture (of course!)—are best left in the hands of professionals. For an idea of the practitioners in your area, check the Yellow Pages (under specific professions, such as acupuncturists, chiropractors, herbalists, homeopaths), ask at churches or community centers, visit a nearby natural-foods store and check bulletin boards for calling cards or ask the manager for suggestions. You'll find additional contact ideas listed under the specific healing alternatives in Part Two.

Important: Check with your physician before stopping or altering any medical regimen.

Step #5: *Plan a Strategy Using Your Health Personality Score*

Now that you understand which alternative healing approach may alleviate the health concerns for which biomedicine isn't well-suited, it's time to plot a strategy. At this point, Glenda might be tempted to take a shortcut. Because several of her health concerns seem appropriate for reflexology or homeopathy or traditional African healing, she might simply locate the appropriate healers in her community and phone them for an appointment.

Why would that be cutting corners? Because it doesn't take into account Glenda's ultimate goal—to Live Wholly. Glenda's Health Personality score is 31—somewhere between Sickness and Wellness. She'll get a lot more out of alternative healing if she documents her health personality on her journey toward Wellness, and eventually Wholeness.

Take Glenda's weight, for instance. Glenda would really like to lose about thirty pounds, and she sees from the Obesity section (p. 294) that nutritional therapy might help her get there. But when she imagines embarking on a new eating plan, all she can think about are years of unsuccessful dieting. And that's discouraging. Glenda sees from her Health Personality score that she tends to be preoccupied with the past (Principle #8: Time focus). Suddenly her fixation on past diet failures makes sense. "I'm gonna turn over a new leaf!" she promises herself. After checking with her doctor, who gives her an enthusiastic green light, Glenda decides to try nutritional therapy—with a small but important difference: she's going to approach it with an eye toward building something positive for the future instead of being stuck in the past. That one attitude adjustment may mean the difference between business as usual and success. On her way to weight loss she might pick up an added bonus—tips for lowering her cancer risk through thoughtful eating.

Hint

When you plan a strategy, you'll find that not all of the sixteen Health Personality principles listed in Table 1 (p. 50) apply to every health concern. Glenda discovered that a preoccupation with the past related to her feelings about weight loss, but the other fifteen Health Personality principles were irrelevant.

Next Glenda turns to her depression, which she suspects could be related to "worriation" over the many emotional and financial concerns faced by all loving single parents. To help her cope, massage therapy looks awfully inviting. What a great way to pamper herself, she thinks. So she decides to take the plunge. Once a week—boy, Friday after work would be ideal!—she'll drop the kids at her cousin's house and head over to a local spa and let someone with golden-smooth hands melt away her cares.

Then Glenda remembers her Health Personality score and thinks about how it applies. Yes, she admits, she is tempted to rely on her massage therapist to take care of her (Principle #4: Source of support). After all, Glenda is in constant demand at home and at work; she's always there for other people, so it's only natural to want someone to return that care and attention, if only for thirty minutes at a time. She sees that moving from Sickness to Wellness means relying less on others and becoming more self-reliant. And then it occurs to her: maybe she can use the techniques she picks up from a masseuse to give herself a sixty-second mini-massage whenever she wants. She can massage her weary legs after a long day of being on her feet, or give her aching hands and wrists a little T.L.C. after an hour or two of nonstop typing. By taking a little more responsibility for her own care, Glenda transforms a once-a-week indulgence into a tool she can use for continuous healing.

Next on the list: hypertension. "Wouldn't it be great if all this massage relaxes me so much that my blood pressure comes down?" Glenda wonders. She makes a mental note to chat with her doctor about this: the massages could mean that she can take less antihypertension medicine, which could help alleviate her "bathroom" problem. In all honesty, Glenda knows that even if her blood pressure falls, her doctor will probably repeat the advice she's heard before: she really needs to start exercising. A regular exercise regimen could lower her blood pressure plus bring so many other benefits—a reduced risk of heart disease, a better blood-cholesterol profile, the list goes on and on. Now, Glenda will tell it to you straight—she has never been a big fan of exercise; running around some ol' gym getting all sweaty has never struck her as fun, not nearly as much fun as hanging out with her kids and playing a game. For a moment, Glenda feels stuck.

Then her eye catches Principle #11 (Community-mindedness). She realizes that she's used to thinking about exercise as a lonely, solitary chore—just as the Sickness model predicts. How could she make exercise less isolating? Maybe if she exercised with her kids! Glenda loves to swim, and her kids love the water. Why not bring them along on regular trips to the public pool? They could even make a game of it, recording their swimming accomplishments (number of laps for Glenda, each new swimming skill for the kids) on a chart that gets taped to the refrigerator. "I'm a genius!" Glenda congratulates herself.

Hint

We often think of alternative healing approaches as substitutes for biomedicine, but they can also supplement it. In Glenda's case, the use of exercise and a healthful diet might enable her to take less antihypertension medicine.

On to Glenda's stomach troubles. Glenda will be the first to admit that she doesn't always listen to what her tummy is telling her. On Saturdays, for example, between all the time she spends plowing through household chores and tending to her kids, she'll sometimes realize as she's putting dinner on the table that she herself hasn't eaten all day.

But her stomach seems to bother her more at work than at home, for some odd reason. Glenda scans the Health Personality chart (Table 1, p. 50). The very first item is Self-connectedness (Principle #1). As she thinks about it, Glenda realizes that she never seems to have an upset stomach on days that her boss is out of the office. And what a boss! He's a racist, sexist, insecure little control freak who gives Glenda confusing, contradictory directives—then berates her for not fulfilling them. The man makes her sick to her stomach—literally. She hasn't noticed the connection before, Glenda realizes, because she's used to thinking about her stomach as separate from the rest of her (the Sickness Approach). Moving to Wellness means becoming more attuned to the mind-body connection—in other words, how her emotions over this hopeless little man affect her stomach.

To help her make that transition to Wellness, Glenda discovers a nice trick. Under the entry to "Stress" in Part Three (p. 314), she finds that aromatherapy offers a quiet, unobtrusive way to calm the spirit. If she keeps a little vial of rose oil in her desk drawer, she can rub a little into her palms and inhale its calming vapors whenever she feels the Neanderthal who signs her paycheck is about to get on her last nerve.

That's how you build your personal strategy to bring you from Sickness to Wellness to Wholeness. You can address any number of health concerns this way. All you have to do is repeat the process explained above. Once you have your Health Personality score (Step #1), and you've asked yourself how well modern medicine is addressing your health concerns (Step #2) so you can identify good candidates for alternative healing methods (Step #3), you simply read through the entries on particular health concerns in Part Three (Step #4) and plan a strategy using your Health Personality score (Step #5).

Hint

Glenda's case shows that there are different ways to plan a strategy. Option #1: Start with a Health Personality item, then think of how it affects a specific health concern. For example, as a person with some Sickness Personality traits, Glenda tended to think of her body as separate from her mind (Principle #1: Self-connectedness). Being aware of that tendency helped her make the connection between emotional stress caused by being around her terrible boss, and her upset stomach.

Option #2: Start with an alternative therapy (like massage, for example) and consider how it might bene t your health concerns. Glenda did that when she focused rst on massage therapy, then looked for ways to apply it. She decided it might help ease her depression, worriation, and hypertension.

Use whatever strategy-building method works for you.

As with everything new, you may find that piecing together an alternative healing strategy feels a bit awkward at first. But expect that; it's natural. The more you practice it, the easier and more natural it will feel. That's why it's important to think of gradual change.

Take it Gradually

If you've ever tried the Grapefruit Diet, the Cabbage Soup Diet, or any other eat-as-much-as-you-want-of-this-single-food-until-you-get-sick-of-it diet, you already know that crash diets are about as successful as the first and final voyage of the *Titanic.* You can only eat but so much cabbage or grapefruit, so the diet ends up reducing the total number of calories you take in. When you restrict your calorie intake drastically, your body thinks you're starving. So it responds by slowing your metabolism, which means you burn calories—and lose weight—progressively more slowly, and eventually not at all. This is why crash diets never work, at least not permanently. When it comes to weight loss, as with any habit change, there's a lot to be said for the gradual approach—making gradual improvements in our diet and exercise habits, in our mental and spiritual outlook, and in how we relate to the world around us. Slow change is lasting change.

Well, "slow and steady" wins all sorts of races. Moving from

Sickness to Wellness to Wholeness takes patience, and it's not an endeavor that you should try to accomplish overnight. But you'd be surprised at the results you can achieve without spending your entire lifetime at it. Andrew Weil, M.D., a Harvard-trained physician and best-selling author who specializes in natural healing, says people can do a lot to discover their inner sense of wholeness and peace in as little as eight weeks. Dr. Weil's program, which he outlines in *Spontaneous Healing* (Alfred A. Knopf, 1995), takes the gradual approach. For example, to improve your diet he recommends eating some fresh broccoli in week one. Well, anyone can do that, right? In week two, he prescribes one serving of fish and a visit to a natural-foods store to try one dish made with soybeans. By the end of the eight weeks, you find yourself feasting on an entirely new range of delicious meals: two weekly meals of fish and two of soy protein, plus heaping servings of whole grains, ginger, garlic, and so forth. But you have hardly noticed the shift because the change is so gradual.

The same trick works for exercise and any other component that you'd like to incorporate into your new healthful lifestyle. Slow and steady. Before you know it, you're enjoying a thoroughly different lifestyle. You're exercising more, eating better, taking time to relax, to refresh, to enjoy the silence. It's a way of being that brings you closer to Whole Living with each passing week.

Try to focus on one change at a time, too. A long laundry list of changes can feel overwhelming. It's better to focus on one new resolution at a time. Once you've got that mastered, you can move on to other items.

Again, don't be dismayed if your feet feel a little wobbly at first. Eventually, the sureness and confidence you're seeking will become second nature.

When Are You Whole Living?

Whole Living isn't like having a baby, or running a 5K race, or washing the dishes—things that have beginnings and endings.

True, there's a starting point—the moment you decide to Live Wholly. But there's no clear-cut end point. Babies are born, an athlete crosses the finish line, the last dish is dried and put away—but there's no magical point at which anyone can definitively say, "I am finally Whole Living." That's because Whole Living is a process. It's an ongoing, evolving state of being.

If you're a goal-oriented person who likes clear-cut boundaries, the idea of having no end point can be a little disconcerting. We're used to thinking about the events in a person's life the same way we think about a straight line. Just as a straight line has a beginning and an end, so, too, do diet makeovers, consultations with herbalists, relaxing baths, exercise plans, visits to iridologists, and other healing projects.

But don't think of Whole Living in terms of a straight line. Think of it as a circle. It's the same distinction that separates how different cultures view life itself. Western cultures—and America is a prime example—think of life as linear: it has a beginning (birth), a middle (adulthood), and an end (death). Traditional cultures—like many in Africa and Asia—think of life as circular. Reincarnation is a perfect example, but you don't have to believe that the dead return in another life form to appreciate how life moves in cycles.

Let's take an example closer to home. As you finish reading this chapter a few minutes from now, you might be curious to learn more about a certain healing technique—say, acupressure. Or maybe you're stuck in bed with a cold, and you wonder what will get you back on your feet again. Before you get a chance to read on, you're interrupted by a phone call. One thing leads to another, and you don't think about this book for a while.

Then one day at church, you overhear two ushers talking about how Sister So-and-So's child recovered from a ferocious chest cold after her mother took her to Miss Judy, a neighborhood herbalist. That reminds you to pick up the book again, which you do once you get home. That afternoon, you take the Health Personality

Quiz and start to piece together a strategy that will move you from Sickness to Wellness.

The strategy works well. You feel positive change in your life, and you begin to experience a sense of renewal and fortification from your work to transform dependence to independence, past living to future living, and interest into involvement. You're happy with this new stage in your life: you feel healthier, stronger, and more vibrant. And because you're content with your newfound health, you relax a bit.

Of course, anything will atrophy if you don't exercise it enough. Over the months, you catch yourself slipping back into some of your old habits. You catch yourself and decide to refer back to your old Health Personality Quiz for a reminder of how to continue your journey to Whole Living.

Each time you renew your efforts to rediscover traditional ways of healing and to incorporate them into your life, you make a full circle. Every time you renew your commitment to live your life in concert with your body's natural rhythms, you refresh your commitment to genuine health. Each time you review your Health Personality score, think about how you live your life, and use alternative approaches for your healing, you move closer and closer to Whole Living.

No One Magic Solution

One of the characteristics of alternative healing is that many roads lead to the same destination. That flexibility is a major distinction between biomedicine and alternative healing systems. It lets you be creative in fashioning a healing approach that works best for you.

Let's say you're a one-pack-a-day smoker. A graceful habit it's not, but you've been going at it for so long that quitting just feels impossible. Your doctor wants you to give it up, and nobody wants to more than you. But all he can recommend is the much-heralded nicotine patch. Yes, you know the patch worked for your brother-in-law, and your ex-smoker next-door neighbor is so enthusiastic about the thing that you figure he ought to up and sign on to be a distributor for the company. But the patch strikes you as costly, cumbersome, and unappealing.

Well, patch or no patch, alternative approaches offer lots of additional ideas that fit not only with your Health Personality score, but also with your overall personality. For instance, if you're good about watching what you slip between your lips, you may benefit from six daily meals of fresh fruits, vegetables, proteins, and whole-grain breads and pastas. This combination keeps blood sugar levels steady, and helps to prevent the food cravings that often mess with smokers during nicotine withdrawal, according to Pavlo Airola, author of *How to Get Well* (Health Plus, 1974).

Using diet to help you kick the habit is one alternative healing approach, but there are others. Maybe you're not Mr. or Ms. Conscientious in the food department. Or maybe your heavy-duty family or job responsibilities mean the six-meal-a-day plan is unworkable. But you do enjoy spending a few minutes of solitude in your garden each evening after dinner is done and the dishes are washed. So why not go to Plan B? Use that time to do a little creative visualization. Studies show that many smokers use tobacco to help them handle anxiety, says Sundar Ramaswami, Ph.D., a clinical psychologist in Stamford, Connecticut, in *New Choices in Natural Healing* (Rodale, 1995). If you meditate, your mind learns another way to relax so you may not have to rely so much on tobacco, he says.

Or there's Plan C. Maybe you've always been the experimental type. A throw-caution-to-the-wind guy or gal. Maybe you would jump at the chance to try something called hydrotherapy—the use of water for healing. Hydrotherapy can help you detoxify your body while you're trying to kick the habit, says Charles Thomas, Ph.D., a physical therapist at California's Desert Springs Therapy Center, in *New Choices in Natural Healing*. It works like this. You take a hot shower, wrap your body in a sheet that's been wrung out with cold water, then lie on a bed and have someone cover you with wool blankets. You'll feel cool at first, but eventually you'll start to sweat as your body heat slowly dries the sheets. Stay wrapped for one to two hours while you perspire. One treatment a day can help you diminish your craving for tobacco, Thomas says.

No one solution works for everyone—which is good, actually, considering how variable people are and how diverse their needs can be. These and many other alternative approaches offer options and answers for real people who are grappling with real health concerns—and they're solutions that are filled with hope.

What's in Store

In Part Two, you'll read about specific alternative healing approaches, from acupressure to vitamin therapy. It describes how each health approach works, the benefits you can expect from it, and any cautions you should bear in mind while pursuing it. This section also covers questions you should ask a practitioner to help you identify an experienced, competent healing professional; the cost of a typical session; and information on using the technique on your own.

Then in Part Three of this book, you'll find information on dozens of health concerns for which alternative healing approaches are often beneficial. Under each listing, you'll see a description of the health concern, information on what can cause it, and a discussion of various alternative approaches that are useful in remedying it. Once you take the Health Personality Quiz, use Part Three to identify ways that you can bring alternative healing methods to bear on health concerns for which biomedicine doesn't seem to be an ideal match.

» PART TWO «

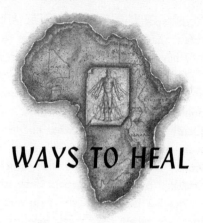

WAYS TO HEAL

To begin to Live Wholly, you need to learn new techniques for healing. This section explores key alternative healing methods, from acupuncture to vitamin and nutrition therapy, that will take you beyond conventional medicine into a whole new world of wellness. Additionally you'll find short stories on things like the healing powers of prayer, meditation, holistic dentistry, bathing, and much more.

We describe each healing method and explain how it works. Then, because no method is foolproof, you'll learn the best uses for the technique as well as cautions to bear in mind. Then you'll find our advice on how to choose a therapist, along with estimated costs of treatment and information on whether you can practice the healing method on your own. Finally, you'll learn where to go for additional information.

Acupressure

"That's it; that's the spot," patients often tell Atlanta, Georgia, acupressurist Yahfaw Shacor. "After clients come to me, they say, 'I thought I would have to live with this pain forever, but now I know I don't.'" During her twenty-plus years of experience with massage and acupressure, Shacor says such expressions of gratitude are not uncommon.

It's not difficult to understand why clients sing Shacor's praises. Acupressure can bring eye-opening relief, often after just a handful of sessions. "I recently worked with someone with sciatica, a condition marked by a shooting pain down the back of one leg. He had developed a limp from the pain and had difficulty sitting or standing," she recalls. Their first meeting lasted for two-and-one-half hours, during which time the acupressurist used heat and ice, as well as vibration and energy therapy to relax the client enough for her to begin neuromuscular work. "When he got up off the table, to his surprise, he could walk without any pain," she recalls. Shacor cautioned her client that while he felt better, he wasn't cured. Sure enough, his pain had returned by the second session. "It really hadn't gone anywhere; it felt better because it was getting better, but it wasn't healed." After the third session, however, he felt so good that she had to phone him to return for the fourth. "To be sure a condition is properly addressed, I like to see patients for a series of six visits initially. The frequency of visits depends on the degree of pain they are in. Usually twice a week for the first two weeks and then once a week for the last two visits is enough." After the six visits, Shacor assesses progress with the client and plans from there. "In many cases, treatment can then go to more preventive care, with a client coming once a month or every two months to make sure the problem doesn't return," she says.

Shacor stresses the importance of preventive care. "Don't wait until you have a problem to come in and have an acupressure session," she says. She advises people to "put the same kind of energy into yourself that you do with your hair and nails or your favorite sports team."

Alice Hiatt, an instructor at the Acupressure Institute in Berkeley, California, describes the results that people get with acupressure as nothing short of amazing. "After just one session, endurance is increased, you feel more energetic, pain subsides," she says. "I live this with every client I have who is willing to let go and receive the benefits."

Letting go can be hard for many African Americans. "Many of us [African Americans] don't understand the benefits of acupressure and other alternative healing methods," Shacor says. "We generally want the insurance company to pay for it, and if it's not covered, we don't bother with it. I always say this: 'You've tried everything else; why not try a little of this?'" Shacor says that African Americans' initial reluctance typically dissolves after the first treatment session. In her experience, they always come back for seconds. "They just have to trust me to touch them. That's all it takes to open the channels and let the energy flow."

"The best possible gift you can give someone is through your hands," says Hiatt, who has taught midwives at the University of Ghana how to use acupressure in childbirth and worked on villagers in Tanzania. She believes the benefits of acupressure stem from the inherent value of touch. "Acupressure works because of your intention to give unconditional love with every point you touch. It's giving from your heart."

What is Acupressure?

Acupressure is similar to acupuncture without needles. Just as in acupuncture, an acupressurist attends to points on the human body that produce a particular effect when pressure is applied. Both methods share the concept that there are fourteen energy pathways (meridians) along which the body's energy or life force—known as *chi* or *Chi* (pronounced "chee")—flows. There are 350 points along the meridians. If points become blocked, then energy, which is said to control the proper functioning of all the organs and cells, cannot flow freely through the body. The inability of the *chi* to flow properly is said to be the source of disease and discomfort.

"Some consider acupressure to be 'do it yourself acupuncture,' " says Joyce Moon, a New York-based acupressurist for fourteen years. "But that's a little too simplistic. Because you don't use needles, acupressure is not as direct at getting at the points of the body as acupuncture is. It is, however, useful on an ongoing basis as a way to prevent illness or help heal it." Similar to acupuncture, acupressure's two prominent effects are pain relief and sedation.

Acupressure can be helpful for people who have a strong aversion to needles. That makes it particularly useful with children. "When a child is traumatized—say he bumped his leg and he's screaming—just apply pressure to points in the top of the head and he will calm down immediately. It's also good for emergencies like a seizure or an asthma attack." Shacor teaches asthmatic children pressure points that relieve a sudden attack.

Moon, who is also a certified acupuncturist, opts to use acupressure with clients who see her less frequently than her regulars. "That way I can teach them the points where they can get relief for themselves from, say, chronic sinusitis, headaches, stomach distress, or tooth pain."

Like many alternative methods, acupressure is tailor-made for self-healing. "This is different from western medicine in which the patient is often dependent on what the physician says. The doctor takes the credit for the healing," Hiatt says. "But in acupressure, we don't heal anyone; people heal themselves."

How Does it Work?
Acupressure points, when given a certain amount of pressure, change the energy flow to create balance within the body. Shacor

cites an example to explain how acupressure works. "Let's say a person comes to me for the painful nerve condition sciatica. I will hold down points along the hip for thirty to sixty seconds or longer, working with the person's breath. As he or she inhales and exhales, I apply and release pressure until I feel the blocked energy begin to move freely." In addition to applying pressure on the points along the hip, Shacor will also work with stomach, bladder, and kidney points. "You have to work along the whole channel in order to bring about balance." Once there is balance in the body, health is restored.

Hiatt stresses that the energy released during acupressure is intangible. "It's electrical, similar to electricity in the air or the energy you feel when you walk into a room. Acupressure appears to work by moving energy from a high place to a low place along the meridian lines."

As with other holistic methods, which by definition examine the whole person (mind, body, spirit) to determine the cause of a particular ailment, an acupressure session begins with the practitioner getting a thorough medical history from the client. "People will come with an issue—be it spiritual, physical, or emotional," Hiatt begins. After taking a medical history, the practitioner begins an assessment. He or she takes vital signs—but not the blood pressure and the pulse in the same way as a western doctor. Western physicians listen to one pulse. "An acupressurist listens to twelve pulses [six on each wrist]; you can tell how each organ is functioning by the quality of the pulse—if it's deep, slow, rapid, or weak." Each of the organ systems is assessed to find the location of the blockages.

In addition to the pulse, acupressurists also examine the color of the eyes and quality of the color of the skin. "There will be tinges of yellow and green in the skin if there is a gallbladder or liver problem," Moon explains. The color of and any coating on the tongue, the brittleness of fingernails and dryness of hands, a person's body odor, the quality of a person's voice and sound of breathing, and the person's chief complaints all help an acupressurist assess a client's condition. "You can't just go by one indication (like a coating on the tongue)," Moon says. "You have to look at the whole person—diet, fingernails, what a person says. All could offer the insight needed to properly assess the situation." Such an examination could take up to two hours.

A client's condition may have an emotional component. "A person might come with a stiff neck—that's the physical problem," Hiatt says. "It could be that the person has a lot of anger and the neck is where they hold the tension." Acupressure addresses both the emotional and the physical. "It's like when you're upset and someone gives you a hug, it helps supports you—you are stronger. That's what we (acupressurists) do; we touch very specific points that help physical, mental, and emotional conditions." In this way, Hiatt stresses, acupressurists are quite unlike many physicians. "We do not diagnose or treat. We assess what's going on and help the body take care of itself."

Best Uses
Acupressure offers relief from a variety of conditions, from tooth pain, headaches, and sinusitis to stress, stomach distress, backaches, and motor recovery after strokes.

Hiatt, a licensed nurse who has combined acupressure with western medicine, reports the common application of acupressure for knee problems, colds, shoulder or neck pain, fatigue and sleeplessness, as well as for heart problems, cancer and AIDS. "Human touch is a powerful healer," she says.

Once a condition has been identified, the acupressurist determines the meridian points to apply pressure. "You have to press hard for fifteen to thirty seconds," Moon stresses. "Make a circular motion around the point to make sure you hit the entire area of the point."

Cautions

Avoid areas with blood clots; applying pressure to a point could cause the blood clot to move, thus causing a potentially life-threatening situation. Avoid working near varicose veins or open injuries. Pressure in such areas can cause intense pain. While pregnant women can receive acupressure, certain points along the stomach should be avoided so as not to induce labor. Long fingernails can break the skin, as can overzealous pressure on the points. Press firmly, but not to the point where the skin is broken or bruised.

If the therapist is reasonably well trained, complications are extremely rare.

Choosing a Therapist

Ask about an acupressurist's training and his or her experience in dealing with your ailment. Be sure to ask about healing methods the practitioner uses in addition to acupressure. For example, Shacor uses deep-tissue massage, visualization, and aromatherapy in her acupressure sessions.

If you are pregnant or have a serious health condition, choose a therapist with plenty of experience. "A student or someone just out of school is not the best choice to work on a person with cancer," Hiatt suggests.

Choose a therapist who speaks your language. Hiatt keeps her explanations simple. "A lot of people are afraid when a therapist says to a client on his or her first visit, 'Just by looking at you, I can tell you everything about you.' Some people don't want you to know everything about them," she says. Also, I'm not going to get into *chi,* meridians, and all that. I'll just say something like 'There seems to be a lot of stress around your knee,' and let them say 'How did you know I had surgery last year?' "

While there is no national certification in acupressure, many therapists are certified in acupuncture, which in some states allows them to practice both methods. Check with individual state governing boards to determine the requirements in your state.

Cost

Acupressure sessions can last from fifteen minutes to two hours. An average cost ranges from $25 to $80 per session, depending on where you live.

Can I Do It Myself?

You can practice acupressure on yourself. An acupressurist can show you self-help techniques for a wide range of health conditions.

For More Information

The Acupressure Institute
1533 Shattuck Avenue
Berkeley, CA 94709
510–845–1059

Relieving Headache, Stress, and Tension with Acupressure

Headaches are believed to result from altered circulation in the head created by dietary, emotional, or physical imbalance. In Chinese medicine it is believed that headaches are the result of an imbalance in the liver and gallbladder. Liver and gallbladder imbalance causes migraine headaches, while stomach and digestive imbalance causes forehead headaches. For relief, dispersion of the stagnant *chi* in both the head and organs must occur to achieve balance. Manipulate the following points:

GB20: Located at the base of the skull in the hairline in the hollow between the front and back neck muscles, behind the bony prominence behind the ear. Administerer should direct pressured movements toward the nose to clear stagnant *chi* in the head.

Yintang: The point in the middle of the forehead, between the eyebrows. Yintang should be gently dispersed by applying fingertip pressure to shift stagnant *chi* and to clear out those cobwebs that often accompany headaches.

St36 and Liv3: St36 is located approximately four finger-widths below the kneecap, outside the tibia. Massage this area to stimulate the digestive system and relieve frontal headaches. Liv3 can be found on the furrow of the top of the foot between the first and second toes where the bones merge. Disperse this point to smooth the flow of *chi*.

STRESS AND TENSION

While some stress may be good for you, too much can prove fatal. In Chinese medicine too much stress or tension equals blocked *chi*, which means energy is not flowing properly throughout the body. To alleviate stress and tension in the body, upper body tension should be directed downward into vital energy. Manipulate the following points:

Liv3: As mentioned above, Liv3 can be found on the furrow of the top of the foot between the first and second toes where the bones merge. Disperse downward to the flow of *chi;* this allows stagnant heat energy in the upper body to descend.

LI4: This point is found in the web between the thumb and index finger on the back of the hand. It should be rubbed to relieve tension in the jaws, neck, and shoulders. It also assists *chi* to descend and clear heat. **This point should never be used during pregnancy.**

GV20: This point is located in the middle of the top of the head, between the ears. Disperse it to clear tension in the head and cloudy thoughts and to raise pure, clear *chi*. For immediate relief, place one drop of Bach Flower Rescue Remedy on this point. **Do not use this point if you suffer from hypertension.**

Acupuncture

One day an elderly patient walked into the office of Houston, Texas, acupuncturist Dard Muhammad, L.Ac., complaining of chronic frozen shoulder. "She couldn't move her shoulder beyond a certain point without extreme pain," recalls Muhammad. Six visits later, the woman could move her arm high enough to reach over her head and touch her opposite ear.

The miracle remedy? Acupuncture, an ancient technique that's among the world's most popular healing systems. "For accelerated healing and the fastest recovery humanly possible, acupuncture is one of the best-kept secrets in conventional and sports medicine," Muhammad says.

Muhammad classifies the woman's complaint as an energy problem, meaning she lacked enough energy to raise her shoulder. "The body is always trying to heal itself. In the woman's case, she didn't have the proper stimulation to lift her shoulder. Acupuncture was successful at clearing the pathway so her energy could flow freely."

Muhammad says acupuncture represents a textbook example of the difference between eastern and western healers. "In eastern

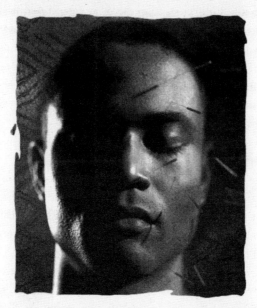

medicine, the practitioner is more like a gardener, nurturing the whole plant—you have to look at the whole person to determine the best way to treat an ailment," he explains. "Western practitioners of conventional medicine are more like mechanics with a cut-it-or-kill-it mentality. Antibiotics and other drugs are used to stomp out a virus or disease. But in eastern medicine, practitioners try to strengthen the body to heal itself."

While acupuncture is traditionally used as preventive care against various ailments, it is also effective for treating existing ailments. But waiting until you're sick is not the most effective way to reap the benefits of this technique. "Black folks have naturally grown up with a skepticism about going to the doctor," says Abayomi Meeks, O.M.D. (Oriental medicine doctor), a Denver, Colorado, acupuncturist. "However, holistic medicine is a practical medicine that is cost-effective and shows results in a brief period of time."

"We have to take an entirely different look at our health,"

says Los Angeles, California, acupuncturist Joseph Acquah, O.M.D. "Chinese medicine is usually used as preventive therapy, but in this country a person usually will not turn to a nontraditional therapy until everything else has failed and they're in dire straits." The best time to see an acupuncturist, he says, is when you are doing well.

What is Acupuncture?

Acupuncture is based on the premise that the body has a network of energy pathways. The energy, known as *chi* or *Chi* (pronounced "chee") in the Chinese tradition (also called ashé in the African tradition and prana in the Indian tradition), flows through these pathways. The *chi* circulates within the body through fourteen invisible energetic paths known as meridians. Most of the meridians connect to one of the major internal organs. The *chi*, or energy, is said to power the organ, enabling it to function properly. "When a person is in a healthy state, energy is flowing smoothly and naturally," Dr. Meeks says. "When disease is present in any form, however, there is imbalance in the pathways, and the *chi* does not flow properly."

There are over 350 specific acupoints on the meridians. Inserting fine acupuncture needles at these points improves the flow of the *chi* in the meridians, restoring balance. "When you introduce anything to the body, it [the body] will ask the question 'Are you friend or foe?' " Muhammad explains. "If foe, the immune system will go into effect and try to suppress the invader. Acupuncture, however, is a friend to the body, helping it to relax and rebalance its energy system."

Acupuncturists describe the energy that flows through the body as electromagnetic. "Acupressure points located along these pathways are points of entry and exit and areas of high electrical potential," explains Dr. Meeks. Metal needles are used as conductors to direct energy through areas of the body where healing is needed. Manipulation of the needles at these points restores balance to the body.

Treatment points are selected on the basis of pulse and tongue diagnosis, examination, observation, and questioning. "Every ailment has different points of entry," Muhammad says. The points affect the meridian system. Very thin needles—most no thicker than a human hair—are inserted on the points and then manipulated by twirling or pumping. "A half turn to the left and a half turn to the right is how I rotate the needles to stimulate the *chi*," Muhammad adds. It has been his experience that such manipulation aids in the removing of blockages and stimulates the flow of energy.

Thus, acupuncture utilizes the body's own recuperative powers to jump-start the body into healing itself. "When any of us breaks our skin, scratches, or cuts ourselves, the body goes into action to heal that spot," Dr. Acquah says. "In acupuncture, we break the skin at specific sites shown to produce healing for a particular ailment." As an example, Dr. Acquah explains that if a person experiences a headache, there is likely to be a sore spot between the thumb and index finger on the back side of the hand. "Pain in that spot is reflective of disease and imbalance," he explains. "Breaking the skin at that location with the insertion of very thin needles relieves the imbalance causing the headache, allowing the *chi* to flow properly."

According to the philosophy behind acupuncture, some diseases operate on the blood level and some operate on the energy level. To holistically treat blood-level diseases (such as cancer or AIDS), you need herbs and proper nutrition in combination with a technique such as acupuncture. For energy-level ailments—which can range from the woman's frozen shoulder to stress or drug abuse—acupuncture is very effective. Muhammad has treated more than 15,000 cases of drug abuse in Houston, Texas. "When the body is engaged in substance abuse, energy systems that affect the kidneys and the liver will be out of balance," he says. "You can address such organ imbalances by stimulating points on the ear that correspond to the kidneys and liver."

How Does it Work?

As with most alternative therapies, the practitioner begins by having clients fill out an intake form. The form informs the acupuncturist of the client's history, as well as what the client hopes to gain from the session. "We look at the whole person, including their lifestyle, spiritual practices, sleeping patterns, and their chief complaints," Dr. Meeks explains. Daily patterns—such as what time the client goes to sleep, if they sweat while asleep, food cravings, and regularity of bowel movements—are also examined.

But acupuncturists do not rely solely on what the client reports. "We also look at the tongue to see if there is any indication of hot, cold, or swelling," Muhammad says. In Chinese medicine, each organ in the body is represented on an area of the tongue. For example a pale red tongue is normal, a red tongue indicates internal heat, while a blue-black tongue signifies internal cold. Such knowledge helps a therapist determine the most effective acupoints.

Acupuncturists also take the client's pulse. Unlike western physicians, an acupuncturist feels for six different pulses on each wrist. The speed, depth, and overall quality of the pulses are all important. Each pulse correlates with a particular meridian and internal organ. Acupuncturists feel the pulse that relates to the heart, gallbladder, kidneys, lungs, liver, and other major organs. "The pulse tells us the balance of energy in the body," Dr. Acquah says. "We not only feel for speed, but strength, how narrow or how wide the pulse is, how deep (how much pressure it takes to feel the pulse) or whether it's right at the surface."

After the intake and examination are complete, the acupuncturist inserts needles along the indicated points. Before insertion, many acupuncturists calm the needle-shy with a demonstration. "Acupuncture needles are not like the needles you get when you go to the doctor," Muhammad explains. "Still, to calm any fears of new clients, I demonstrate by inserting a needle on their hand to show that there really is only a small and quick pinch when the needle is inserted. No extreme pain and no blood." Such a demonstration calms the fears of first-timers.

"It feels like what you feel when you pluck a hair," Muhammad says. Dr. Acquah says clients typically report any of five different sensations: tingling under the skin, numbness, a hitting-the-funny-bone sensation, a dull ache, or swelling or heaviness. "These are good signs that say you are getting the optimal effect of your treatment."

Acupuncture needles are made of stainless steel, silver, or gold. "The needles are either disposable or marked, sterilized, and kept specifically for a particular client," Dr. Meeks explains. Once the needles are inserted, the client remains with the needles in place for twenty to forty minutes while the body begins to respond. During a session, only the areas of the body where the needles are inserted need to be exposed. "To treat headaches, there is no disrobing at all," Dr. Acquah says. "For the back, a client may need to remove upper garments."

Bleeding is rare, occurring in fewer than 5 percent of clients, Dr. Acquah says. "Because of the effort to avoid blood vessels, arteries and veins, plus the thinness of the needle, any minute puncture seals itself."

After a session, most people feel relaxed and may see results immediately. "I recommend that clients who are suffering from an acute or painful condition come at least twice a week," Dr. Meeks says. "For most people, fewer than ten treatments is sufficient, but the younger the ailment, the shorter the course of treatment." To treat a chronic ailment or disease, fifteen to twenty treatments are recommended. "In less than five treatments, you should know whether acupuncture is helping you," he adds.

Best Uses

The science behind acupuncture is unclear, but the experiences of acupuncturists and their clients indicate that it is effective for preventing and healing many ailments. In fact, acupuncture is so effective against particular ailments that the World Health Organization lists 100 diseases for which it is effective. "Bursitis, gastritis, arthritis, rheumatism, constipation, diarrhea, ulcers, hypertension, reproductive disorders, the flu and respiratory problems such as asthma and bronchitis, and pain are all helped or even cured with acupuncture," Dr. Acquah reports. "Acupuncture is also an immune-system enhancer, and while it is not a cure by itself for cancer or AIDS, it can relieve the side effects of the toxic drugs used to treat such conditions." Acupuncture is also effective at reducing fever and lowering blood pressure.

Cautions

Acupuncture is safe for most common ailments, but should only be practiced by a qualified practitioner. There is minimal risk of contracting communicable diseases if you consult a registered practitioner who uses proper hygiene and sterilization or uses disposable needles.

"Don't have a full stomach when treated, but neither should you feel totally empty," Dr. Meeks says. "You should be comfortable and not completely exhausted." Dr. Meeks also says that women in their third trimester of pregnancy should consult a physician before receiving acupuncture. "Also, the use of alcohol, drugs, coffee, or nicotine immediately after treatment nullifies any positive effects you may have achieved. Remember the purpose of seeking acupuncture is to promote healing. Placing toxins in your body runs counter to what acupuncture is trying to do."

Choosing a Therapist

Training is key. "Some physicians take a 100-hour course and think they are acupuncturists," Dr. Acquah says. While there is currently no national license for acupuncturists, practitioners can be certified through the National Commission for the Certification of Acupuncturists and each state requires acupuncturists to obtain a license before they can practice. So ask about an acupuncturist's training.

Before beginning a session, ask about any aspects of acupuncture that make you uneasy ("Will it hurt?" "Will I bleed?") "The acupuncturist should encourage the client to ask as many questions as necessary in order to feel comfortable," according to Muhammad.

It is also important to ask a therapist about his or her philosophy on healing. "How will a therapist treat you?" Dr. Meeks explains, "Do you want to see a practicing physician who will treat you with acupuncture and still prescribe medicine, perhaps before giving the treatment a chance to work?"

Ask what type of needles the acupuncturist uses. "Disposable needles are best," Dr. Meeks advises. "If the needles are not disposable, find out how the needles are cleaned."

Ask the acupuncturist how much experience they have with your particular ailment. Also find out what other techniques—such as reflexology, aromatherapy, or massage—your practitioner knows so you have an idea of the range of treatment you can expect.

After a session, a good acupuncturist should be able to offer advice on how to maintain the benefits of the session. "Your acupuncturist should tell you types and amount of exercise, things to avoid—such as foods, drafts, and heat—suggest breathing exercises, and make you aware of patterns you may have to break," Dr. Acquah says. Most acupuncturists should also be familiar with herbs and be able to suggest herbs that might assist in your healing.

Cost

A typical session lasts thirty to sixty minutes, but might be briefer for children, the elderly, and the very ill or otherwise injured. The average cost ranges from $40 to $75.

Can I Do It Myself?

Because acupuncture requires a high degree of skill and training, no one except a licensed practitioner should practice it. "It is a simple medicine in its procedure and application, but it is complex to know when to use acupuncture, how to put the needles in, and where to put them," Dr. Acquah says. "The insertion of the needles is very dangerous, points are needled in a certain way, and the therapist must know the contraindications."

To locate a qualified acupuncturist, contact a professional organization (listed below) or seek a referral from friends and family.

For More Information

National Commission for the Certification of Acupuncturists
P.O. Box 97075
Washington, D.C. 20090–7075
Tel: 202–232–1404
Fax: 202–462–6157

American Association of Acupuncture and Oriental Medicine
4101 Lake Boone Trail, Suite 201
Raleigh, NC 27607
919–787–5181

National Acupuncture and Oriental Medicine Alliance
P.O. Box 77511
Seattle, WA 98177–0531
Tel: 206–524–3511

Chinese Medicine

Chinese medicine is made up of a vast system of health care practices and disciplines that have existed for centuries. Its origins can be traced back to the sixth century B.C. to Lao-tzo, who founded Chinese medicine along with Taoism. Lao-tzo believed that optimal health was the result of a balance of opposite and complementary forces, or yin and yang. He also believed that if there is a disruption of *Chi* or *chi*, the vital energy force that flows through the body through energy points or meridians, sickness and disease would prevail. *Chi* is the cornerstone of Chinese medicine. Chinese medicine focuses on prevention as well as treatments of many ailments, and its therapies encompass diagnosis, therapy, terminology and understanding of human physiology and how the body works.

Therapies are used to restore *chi*, or balance, in the body. Some therapies of Chinese medicine are common to many of us, like massage and meditation, herbal remedies and acupuncture, while others, like Chigong, moxibustion and cupping are less familiar. Chigong is a series of breathing exercises combined with meditation that, when used properly, balance and strengthen *chi*. There are two forms of Chigong, internal and external. In internal Chigong, the patient focuses on movement of his or her own *chi*, while external Chigong involves the transfer of *chi* from a master to another person by touch or close proximity. Moxibustion is the process of burning a ball of herbs or Chinese mugwort. The leaves are burned directly onto the body in the location where *chi* is believed to be unbalanced. The heat generated by this process is believed to restore balance and promote healing. Cupping shares some similarities with moxibustion, except that instead of using burning leaves, energy is directed to a specific area of the body by suction. Suction is created by warming the air inside of a glass jar and then placing the jar on the patient's body. Once heat is applied, the body will begin to warm, causing dampness to dissipate and restore *chi*. Cupping is widely recommended for bronchial congestion and other ailments that benefit from direct stimulation like arthritis.

Chinese medicine also operates under the premise that the five elements—fire, earth, metal, water, and wool—are central to treatment and diagnosis of ailments. Practitioners rely heavily on the system of elements to administer treatment to patients. In addition to the elements, the system of pulse taking is also widely practiced. Instead of simply listening to a patient's heart rate, practitioners also listen to the pulse of the other organs to determine their function and balance.

WHAT IT CAN DO FOR YOU

There are many benefits of Chinese medicine. Its longevity as a method of healing is a testimony to that. The elderly and patients suffering from arthritis or cancer can gain relief from their ailments through the use of acupuncture and Chigong. Both exercises enhance balance and muscle tone. Massage and meditation are widely used to lower anxiety and increase relaxation.

For more information:

American Association of Acupuncture and Oriental Medicine
4104 Lake Boone Trail
Suite 201
Raleigh, NC 27607
(919) 787–5181

The American Foundation of Traditional Chinese Medicine
505 Beach
San Francisco, CA 94133

American Oriental Bodywork Therapy Association
Glendale Executive Park
1000 White Horse Road, Suite 510
Voorhees, NJ 08043
(609) 782–1616

Meridians and How They Work

Meridians originate from ancient Chinese medicine, specifically acupuncture. They are the fourteen main channels of energy or life force that run throughout the body and head. Of the fourteen meridians, twelve are bilateral, meaning these points exist on both sides of the body. The remaining two meridians are unilateral and run along the midline of the body. Each meridian is said to affect a particular organ or body system. Meridians, or channels, are used in acupressure and acupuncture to access the more than 300 acupoints throughout the body.

Aromatherapy

Nanikha Sims will tell you point blank about the amazing power of your sense of smell. "In the three years since I have seriously studied and practiced aromatherapy, I have seen muscles relax, complexions clear up, and bodies twisted for years straighten out," says Sims, a Westchester County, New York, aromatherapist. She describes a woman who came to her after unsuccessfully seeking conventional treatment for scoliosis (curvature of the spine). The patient couldn't sit straight and was experiencing swelling. Sims describes that after applying certain oils to the painful areas, the swelling subsided and she experienced tremendous relief after only one treatment.

But physical healing is just one benefit of aromatherapy. The technique is also used for emotional or mental imbalances, as aromatherapist L'dia Muhammad discovered. Muhammad's teenage daughter was what she calls "high strung." "She would always argue with her sister and it was hard to please her," says Muhammad, a midwife in Berkeley, California. Her solution? "An hour before she woke up, I would scent her bedroom air with a few drops of soothing chamomile. Instead of waking up with an attitude, she woke up singing."

Abena Asantewaa, Ph.D., a clinical psychologist and aromatherapist in South Bend, Michigan, uses essential oils to bring about a similar effect. "People come to me for counseling," she says. "We discuss what's going on in their lives, and I suggest a

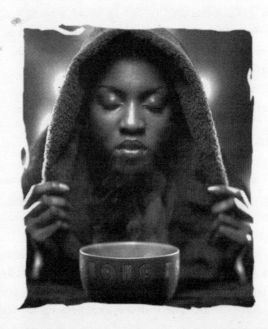

particular oil or blend one for them based on their needs. People can most effectively use a blend that relaxes them; when you are relaxed, energy is released, making people better able to participate in solving their problems."

Whether to relax, to stimulate, or to introduce euphoria, essential oils have a variety of uses, all designed to restore balance to a stressed body, mind, and spirit.

What is Aromatherapy?

Aromatherapy is the use of oils extracted from plants and flowers (often called "essential oils") to alleviate illness. Essential oils typically contain vitamins, antibiotics, and hormones. Once absorbed by the skin, they can be carried throughout the body via the circulatory system.

"Because oils are extracted from plants, the oils contain whatever medicinal properties the plant contains," Asantewaa explains. "Our sense of smell is one of our most underdeveloped senses. Any way you can incorporate fragrances into your life will make you feel better."

Different essential oils have different effects. Chamomile and lavender relax, while rosemary, cinnamon, and peppermint stimulate. And sandalwood, rose, and citrus oils produce euphoria. Essential oils alleviate various health conditions, strengthening the internal organs, boosting the immune defenses, but mostly by relaxing the body. Relaxation returns the body to a balanced state. "A balanced mind, body, and spirit is the goal of aromatherapy," Muhammed says. "It's where good health is maintained."

Aromatherapy is an ancient practice. "Oils from plants, flowers and trees have been discovered in ancient tombs," Sims explains. "And when the bottles were opened, the oils were still fragrant after thousands of years." Because of their antiseptic and antifungal properties and their ability to stop tissue decomposition, essential oils were used to embalm the dead. Among the oils in wide use during ancient times were frankincense, myrrh, cedarwood, onion, garlic, and cypress.

Before distillation, the modern method of extracting essential oils from plants, ancient cultures took advantage of the healing properties of essential oils through a process called smoking. In smoking, depending on a person's ailment, specific plants were thrown into a fire to create smoke, which the patient inhaled. Essential oils were also blended into fatty ointments or pastes, used as antiseptics for wounds and illnesses, and used as deodorants.

The father of modern aromatherapy is René-Maurice Gattefossé, a chemist born in Grasse, France, where essential oils have been extracted for many years for use in cosmetics. During the early 1920s, Gattefossé worked in an essential oils factory. When his hand was badly burned during an explosion in his laboratory, he submerged it immediately in lavender oil. When the wound healed rapidly without infection or scarring, it confirmed for him the healing properties of essential oils. Gattefossé, who is credited with coining the term "aromatherapie," published his findings in a 1928 book by that name.

It was not until World War II when Jean Valet, a French physician, used the antiseptic and antibiotic properties of essential oils to treat injured soldiers, that aromatherapy gained further attention. The publication of Valet's 1964 book, *Aromathérapie,* saw increased focus on the medicinal use of essential oils. Aromatherapy has begun to make inroads into the United States, although the technique has yet to reach the level of acceptance as in France, where aromatherapy is taught in medical schools and dispensed in pharmacies. Many Americans first learn about aromatherapy through massage therapists and reflexologists, many of whom routinely use essential oils to help their clients relax.

How Does it Work?
Aromatherapy invokes the science of smell. When you inhale an essential oil, scent organs in the nose carry specific nerve messages

to brain tissue known as the olfactory bulb. These messages have immediate effects throughout the nervous system, causing stimulation, sedation, or other effects.

But there is another way to receive the beneficial effects of aromatherapy: the oils can be applied to the skin. Rubbing essential oils into the soles of the feet is particularly effective. "The oils penetrate the skin and are absorbed directly into the bloodstream," Sims says. Aromatherapists say the effects of a single such use of essential oils typically linger for up to a week to ten days. Adding six to twelve drops to your bathwater is also effective. The hot water opens the pores, allowing the oils to be absorbed.

Air diffusion is also popular, although it allows lower levels of oils to enter the body because they are so diluted. Air diffusers like aroma lamps (not actually a lamp, but a small container that holds a few drops of oil above a lit candle) and potpourri steamers (both available at health food or new age stores) both spread the aroma of an essential oil into the air. The oils are so concentrated that you can even put a few drops on a cotton ball, put it in a plastic freezer bag and take it out and sniff it throughout the day.

Best Uses

Essential oils are typically used to induce relaxation. As a midwife, Muhammad uses lavender and jasmine to relax women during labor. Inhaling these oils helps calm a woman so she can breathe more deeply. "This way women don't have to rely as much on drugs to relieve pain," says Muhammad, herself the mother of five children. "I massage the oils on her stomach or back or wherever she is feeling pain." For women with high blood pressure, Muhammad rubs ylang ylang on the feet. If a woman's contractions are slow in coming, she uses clary sage, which helps induce contractions.

For digestion problems, Sims recommends tarragon. "Assume you ate something that was not digested well, and it is causing nausea or burping. You can just inhale a little tarragon oil, rub a little on your stomach, or put it on the bottom of your feet," Sims explains.

Peppermint, with its slightly analgesic effect, is good for food poisoning, nausea, cholic, diarrhea, minor or temporary headaches, and travel sickness. "Lemon oil is a good mental stimulant," Muhammad adds. "You could mix it with rosemary to help you stay alert to study for a test." Eucalyptus, that familiar aroma in cough drops, is good for allergy or sinus problems.

Other essential oils are used to relieve anger, reduce stress, build the immune system, reduce swelling, relieve exhaustion, soothe the spirit, and calm insecurities, nightmares, or mood swings.

While each oil has specific qualities, aromatherapists typically use two or three oils blended in tandem to produce a synergistic effect. Blends include citrus and clove oils to prevent infection; eucalyptus and sandalwood oils for a cold or flu; jasmine and ylang ylang oils to calm stressful emotions in a relationship; and tea tree and lemon oils to enhance the immune system. "Blending is where the art of aromatherapy comes into play" explains Muhammad. "Oils like sandalwood and myrrh are like your bass notes, while lemon and lavender are your high notes. Finding just the right blend can help you make beautiful music and create a unique scent just right for you and your needs."

Cautions

Because essential oils are very potent, certain types such as peppermint or cinnamon and some citrus oils can burn or otherwise irritate the skin. Some oils can be toxic. Sims recalls a patient with an earache who was advised to put a drop of a particular oil on a piece of cotton and then put the cotton in her ear. "Instead, the woman dropped the oil directly into her ear. She ended up burning her eardrum." In fact, recommends Muhammad, "Laven-

der and tea tree oil are the only oils that can be used undiluted."
When rubbed on the skin and feet, it is important to dilute other
essential oils with a carrier oil, such as almond, canola, soybean,
or grapeseed oils. Olive oil has a distinctive aroma, so many users
avoid it. As a rule of thumb, add eight to ten drops of essential
oil to two tablespoons of the carrier oil.

While some oils can be taken internally, do so only under the
supervision of a qualified practitioner. Other oils can have even
catastrophic effects. "Lemon oil taken internally could kill you,"
Muhammad says. Carefully follow the directions on the bottle and
respect the guidance of an aromatherapist or authoritative books
on aromatherapy. Like all potent medicines, keep essential oils out
of the reach of children.

If you are pregnant, consult an aromatherapist or authoritative
book on aromatherapy before using any essential oil. While most
oils are safe for use in pregnancy, some—such as pennyroyal, rosemary, juniper and hyssop—can cause abortion or induce prema-
ture labor.

To receive the greatest benefits, select high-quality oils. Beware
of "fragrance oils"—such as those oils you can buy on the street
or even in health food stores. They may be synthetic versions of
essential oils. "The oils should be natural, not synthetic," Dr.
Asantewaa advises. "Synthetic oils may smell appealing, but they
can be ineffective or produce toxic effects like headaches and nausea." One way to tell whether an oil is natural is its price tag. "If
you pay $3 or $4 for a bottle of lavender, chances are you have
lavender cut with less expensive ingredients," Sims says. "The
purer the oil, the more it costs." High-quality essential oils can
range from $15 to $100 a bottle, depending on the oil. For example, citrus oils, which are easily extracted from fruits, cost less
than rose oil, because it takes two tons of rose petals to make one
ounce of pure oil. "Some oils may be expensive, but for the genuine article, it's worth it," Muhammad adds. "A little goes a long

way." "Essential oils should have some texture when you rub it between your fingers, not like an alcohol feel," Dr. Asantewaa says.

Finally, when using aromatherapy (whether on your own or in a session, which usually includes another therapy such as reflexology or massage), drink at least six to eight glasses of water daily. "The oils help to release toxins that have built up in your body," Sims explains. "It's important to drink a lot of water so that those toxins can move out of your system."

Questions to Ask

There is currently no national certification for aromatherapists. To be sure that the practitioner you choose is qualified to guide you through the use of essential oils and to advise you on your particular problem, inquire about the healer's training and experience.

As with other healing methods, the therapist should have you fill out an intake form before treatment asking about your lifestyle and medical history. These questions are designed to give the practitioner an idea of which oils will be most effective for your individual needs.

Choosing a Therapist

In addition to asking about training and experience, intuition can be an important guide. "What do you feel when you meet the practitioner?" Sims says. "If you have a good feeling about a person's energy, rely on those feelings; they are rarely wrong."

Cost

Most aromatherapy sessions last thirty to ninety minutes, depending on whether the treatment is combined with massage, reflexology, or other techniques, which is usually the case because many aromatherapists are certified in those areas. Typical sessions cost $25 to $80. The number and type of oils used often affect the price of the session. Many aromatherapists try to keep sessions inexpensive to appeal to as many people as possible. Low prices are especially important since aromatherapy is not covered by most insurance plans.

Can I Do it Myself?

With an abundance of books and courses on the subject, aromatherapy can be learned easily by virtually anyone.

For More Information

American Aromatherapy Association
P.O. Box 3679
South Pasadena, CA 91031
818–457–1742

International Federation of Aromatherapists
Stamford House
2–4 Chiswick Highroad
London
W41TH, UK
011–44–81–742–2605

Aromatherapy Alphabet

Listed below are several common scents and their healing properties. Many oils are very potent and could cause harm if used improperly. Also, many oils can prove harmful to pregnant women, and should be used under the direction of a physician or licensed aromatherapist only.

Angelica: Stimulates the production of gastric juices, aids digestion; stimulates the production of urine; strengthens the immune system; relieves coughing, helps to expel mucus, used for bronchitis, asthma, colds and flu; strengthens the nervous system.

Basil, French: Soothes the stomach; used to treat constipation; flatulence, nausea, food poisoning; decongests the liver and stimulates bile production; relieves menstrual cramps and promotes the production of menstrual blood; improves circulation; reduces muscular tension and pain; is commonly used to treat rheumatism, arthritis and muscular aches; also clears the mind and improves memory; aids in concentration; soothes fears and helps to combat anxiety, depression and insomnia.

Bergamot: Aids in digestion; stimulates the production of urine; used for flu, tonsillitis, laryngitis, sore throat and bronchitis; helps relieve anxiety, depression and ease grief and sadness; corrects emotional imbalances and increases alertness.

Cade: Used primarily for disorders of the skin like dermatitis, eczema and dandruff. Relieves itching and can be used for mosquito bites. Also an antiseptic and a pain reliever.

Canadian Balsam: Relieves constipation; is used for relief of hemorrhoids; can be used as a laxative and diuretic; used also for respiratory infections like asthma and bronchitis. Assists in healing burns, wounds, and scars. Used as a tonic and a sedative; used to alleviate depression and nervous tension.

Chamomile: Stimulates digestion, tones the stomach and the liver and improves appetite; stimulates the production of urine and menstrual blood; relieves cramps and premenstrual syndrome (PMS); relaxes muscles and relieves pain of arthritis, inflamed joints and sprains; strengthens the immune system; conditions hair; promotes healing of scarred skin tissue; aids in the healing of wounds; used for acne and many other skin disorders. Acts as an antidepressant recommended for irritability and oversensitivity, restlessness and anxiety; improves memory.

Citronella: Tones the stomach, aids digestion, improves appetite; tones the kidneys and stimulates the flow of urine and menstrual blood; used for oily skin and excessive perspiration; is a deodorizer, insect repellent and reduces fever.

Eucalyptus: Stimulates the production of urine, cleans the blood, lowers blood sugar, improves circulation; stimulates respiration, relieves coughing, expels mucus and treats respiratory illnesses such as asthma and bronchitis; reduces fever; helps wounds heal; used also for burns, cuts, blisters; stimulates the mind, relieves inability to concentrate, alleviates mood swings and temper tantrums.

Fennel: Aids digestion, relieves constipation; eases cramps; helps alleviate menopausal symptoms and dissolves kidney stones; helps alleviate respiratory ailments; stimulates skin circulation; used for dull skin, wrinkles, bruises, and cellulitis; improves lactation.

Geranium: Used for diarrhea; stimulates the production of urine, used to treat the urinary tract. Balances hormones during menopause; diminishes water retention during PMS; improves circulation; used for various skin disorders including dry or excessively oily skin; helps heal wounds; combats stress and depression; reduces breast enlargement; lowers blood sugar.

Ginger: Relaxes stomach muscles, tones stomach; used to treat varicose veins and cellulitis; increases mental alertness; improves memory. Is used for debility and nervous exhaustion.

Helichrysum: Stimulates bile production; tones the liver; alleviates spleen and liver congestion; used to relieve muscular aches and pains from sprains and rheumatism; relieves most respiratory ailments; strengthens the immune system; used to treat many skin ailments like acne and dermatitis.

Jasmine: Stimulates the production of gastric juices; tones the uterus, treats dysmenorrhea and many uterine disorders, relieves menstrual cramps, aids in childbirth; treats many muscular and respiratory ailments like laryngitis and muscular sprains; acts as a sedative, soothes and relaxes; helps heal wounds; relieves dry skin.

Lavender: Stimulates digestive system; treats nausea, colic and diarrhea; lowers blood pressure; tones and soothes the heart; calms palpitations; reduces muscular tension; relieves respiratory infections; heals wounds and rejuvenates the skin; treats acne, psoriasis and wrinkles; calms, refreshes and relaxes; treats some mental illnesses like manic depressive illness. Helpful in treating addictions.

Lemon Oil: Stimulates the digestive system; tones the liver and the kidneys; lowers the blood pressure; lowers blood sugar and removes toxins from the blood; aids in treatment of arthritis and rheumatism; stops bleeding; relieves acne and dandruff; exfoliates the skin and enlivens the complexion. Clears the mind, improves concentration and memory. Helps to combat depression, bitterness, irrational fears, and mental blocks.

Melissa: Stimulates the production of gastric juices, tones the stomach and improves appetite; used for asthma to slow breathing and relax respiratory muscles; lowers blood pressure; is a sedative; relieves stress, tension, irritability; combats fever.

Myrrh: Stimulates the digestive system, tones the digestive system; treats diarrhea and loss of appetite; treats hemorrhoids; stimulates the production of white blood cells; improves circulation; treats chapped and cracked skin.

Peppermint: Alleviates nausea caused by sea or travel sickness; helps break up gallstones; aids in treating diarrhea; relieves itching; treats acne and dermatitis; stimulates circulation; treats dry, dull skin; treats mental fatigue and migraine headaches; strengthens the nervous system; alleviates stress.

Rose: Improves and regulates the appetite; aids digestion,

relieves constipation, tones the stomach, liver and spleen; stimulates the flow of bile; treats liver congestion, nausea and ulcers. Is a cleansing agent; gently stimulates the production of menstrual blood; tones and cleanses the uterus. Treats uterine disorders, irregular menstruation and cramps; tones the heart and regulates its action; expels toxins from the blood. Treats respiratory illnesses like asthma, hay fever, and coughs. Combats stress, insomnia, and headaches. Is an aphrodisiac.

Sandalwood: Relaxes digestive muscles; is used to treat genitourinary infections; mild pain reliever; used as a sedative; treats nervous tension, stress, anxiety and depression.

Tea Tree: Used to alleviate intestinal infections; treats fungal infections, thrush, vaginitis, cystitis; treats respiratory infections and illnesses; stimulates the immune system; useful in oral hygiene; relieves gingivitis, mouth ulcers, periodontal disease, and toothaches.

Ylang-Ylang: Relaxing and soothing to the genitourinary tract; helps treat menstrual cramps and PMS; regulates and lowers blood pressure, used for hypertension; used for skin disorders including eczema and acne; combats nervous tension, depression and insomnia.

Chiropractic

In 1895, an unnamed Black office janitor in Davenport, Iowa, found himself in a room with Daniel David Palmer, a grocer and mystic healer. Palmer had a hunch that he could help the janitor, who was deaf. Sure enough, he was right. By manipulating his patient's upper back, where he believed the cause of deafness was located, Palmer was able to restore the janitor's hearing. And in that one seemingly miraculous moment, chiropractic (Greek for "hands-on") was created, and Palmer would forever be known as its father.

Today there are more than 50,000 chiropractors in the United States, making chiropractic the most popular of all alternative healing methods. But despite the therapy's popularity, it has not been without its share of controversy. "I remember back in 1979 when I was in school, there was a so-called chiropractor who gave people adjustments over the phone," recalls Johari Amini Hudson, D.C., an Atlanta, Georgia–based chiropractor of twelve years. "It was a bogus hokus-pokus treatment." Such false claims have plagued the profession for years.

But most of the threat has come from outside of the profession. "The feud against chiropractic therapy was spawned by medical professionals who simply disliked competition," says A. Rush Robinson, D.C., a Memphis, Tennessee–based chiropractor. "Both

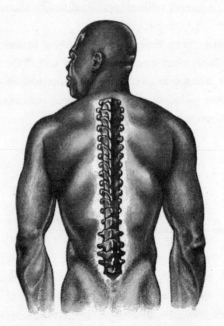

mainstream medicine and chiropractic developed around the same time during the late 1800s, and since then until recently, the medical establishment has led a longstanding smear campaign against chiropractors. Public demand for alternative ways for staying healthy has prodded the medical establishment to become more open to working with chiropractors by referring patients to us."

As for the quacks? With required five-year, postgraduate training at chiropractic schools around the country, a national board examination, and state board examinations in all fifty states, chiropractors have worked hard to elevate the profession.

Although the first chiropractic patient was a Black man, many African Americans know little about the field. "By and large, we [African Americans] have not availed ourselves to chiropractic care due mainly to two historic reasons: a lack of access and a hesitance to try something new," Dr. Robinson explains. "Black doctors tend to take care of Black patients. Black chiropractors make up only 1 percent of the profession, which makes it difficult to find an African American provider, unless you live in a major city."

For Dr. Hudson, increasing the popularity of chiropractic among African Americans is all about education. "Some African Americans who have had sports injuries or car accidents have gone to see a chiropractor," she explains. "Most are surprised to find out that we not only treat lower back pain, but we also have a nutritional approach to diabetes or high blood pressure; we look at the whole person and make suggestions for overall wellness. Educating African Americans about the diversity of ailments and conditions we treat ultimately gets more of them into our offices and on the road to optimal health."

What is Chiropractic?

In chiropractic theory, the nervous system plays a key role in maintaining balance and well-being. The body functions as a result of electrical impulses that descend from the brain down the spinal cord and then to every muscle and gland in the body, controlling and coordinating them. Chiropractors analyze the structure and flexibility of the spine, identifying areas where vertebrae have moved out of alignment.

If one or more vertebrae moves out of alignment, the nerves that exit the spinal column between vertebrae can become pinched. "This alters the electrical impulses traveling from the nerves to various organs and glands. Altering the impulses could cause malfunctions in those organs and glands," says Alfred Davis Jr., D.C., a Montclair, New Jersey-based chiropractor of 16 years. Chiropractors seek to return the body into balance by using their hands to manipulate the spine and other joints and muscles, allowing the neuromusculoskeletal (brain, muscles, and skeleton) system to function smoothly.

"Chiropractic is the science and art of adjusting and manipulating the spinal joints to restore proper function and to relieve nerve pressure to the body," according to Dr. Robinson. "Joints that have lost their proper mobility become locked. Once you lose motion in the human body, we call that death; losing motion to a joint is like the death of that joint—it will not receive its proper nutrition and will eventually become very painful." Full function and balance can be restored, chiropractors argue, through proper manipulation.

A fall, an injury, an accident, poor posture, hereditary weakness, or repetitive activity can cause a vertebra to move out of place. "Physicians might prescribe a pill or give an injection to deaden the pain, but this only eliminates the symptom. Chiropractors try to identify the cause of the problem. If you can get rid of the cause, you can get rid of the symptoms," according to Dr. Davis. In theory, chiropractors believe that virtually all discomfort and disease begin as a result of a misalignment in the spine. Correcting the alignment of vertebrae can bring about relief of pain and discomfort and return the body to a healthy balance.

How Does it Work?

The chiropractor examines the spine, looking for irregularities or misaligned vertebrae that may interfere with the functioning of the bundle of nerves inside the vertebrae. "There are twenty-four movable vertebrae along the spine, each one corresponding to different organs," says Dr. Davis. The condition of the patient and where he or she might be experiencing discomfort will be determined by which vertebra is out of alignment. Once identified, the chiropractor attempts to readjust vertebrae that are interfering with nerve function and causing pain.

When chiropractors first see a patient, they take a thorough medical history. They conduct a physical examination, a posture analysis, and a range of motion test to try to locate a specific tissue or joint causing the problem. They may use x-rays or refer the patient for more specific tests, such as orthopedic or neurological exams, or blood work.

Whatever tests are given, the chiropractor carefully reviews the results with the patient. In some instances, depending on the findings of the test, the chiropractor may opt not to work on the patient. "A patient may have a fractured vertebra," Dr. Hudson explains. "But if the x-ray shows that he or she has a history of cancer, I would refer the person to an oncologist [cancer specialist]. Or if the test determines that the pain is not from a structural problem but a problem with the kidneys, then I would refer the patient to a nephrologist [kidney specialist]."

Once the patient's questions have been discussed, the practitioner begins the chiropractic adjustment to realign the vertebrae. The patient lies facedown or faceup on a table. Using the hands, the chiropractor adjusts vertebrae with a mild thrust. To most people, the procedure is not painful but in fact brings pain relief. "The misaligned vertebra causes more pain than does the thrust to move it back into place," Dr. Hudson explains.

"Chiropractic therapy looks at the structure of the body as a whole," Dr. Robinson says. "Correct the structure, and you correct the function."

Best Uses

"Every medical condition is not a chiropractic problem, but many are," Dr. Hudson says. "Any condition having to do with lower back or neck pain or pains that radiate from the back into the arms or legs can be helped by a chiropractor," Dr. Robinson says. "I have had patients scheduled for lower back surgery who had seen an orthopedic specialist, a neurologist, and a neurosurgeon, all of whom had recommended surgery. Through chiropractic therapy, they were able to avoid it." One of Dr. Robinson's patients had suffered pain in the back and legs for two years and came to him a few days before he was to have surgery. After only three treatments, the patient's pain was relieved and the surgery cancelled.

Dr. Robinson attributes such misdiagnosis by conventional doctors to a less-than-thorough examination and a failure of the specialists to listen to the patient. "The patient's x-ray showed that there was a bulging disk in the lower back. The patient kept telling the doctors that his pain was coming from one place, but the doctors all said it had to be coming from another—the bulging disk." A more thorough examination showed the patient had a misaligned vertebra along the lower back. Once corrected, the disk problem went away.

Chiropractic therapy is also used to treat allergies, asthma, shoulder pains, and work-related injuries. Chiropractors have had success in correcting scoliosis, headaches, and even bed wetting. "Many children who are bed wetters may not have weak bladders or kidney problems," according to Dr. Hudson. "They simply need a lower back adjustment to correct the pinching of nerves in the lower back." Sciatica, osteoarthritis, and osteoporosis are other ailments for which chiropractic has been particularly effective. Some chiropractors claim success at treating heart disease, prostate and impotency problems, epilepsy, and cancer.

Some chiropractors do not limit their work to spinal manipulations. "In Illinois, California, and New York, chiropractors can deliver babies and perform some internal examinations, such as rectal exams," according to Dr. Hudson. "In Georgia, chiropractors give health certificates to people who need to demonstrate to their employer that they are capable of working a particular job."

Even though a patient may seem healthy, many chiropractors recommend a regular (twice a year) check-up. "Preventive care is very important," Dr. Hudson says. "While you may not currently feel any symptoms from a problem, that does not mean the potential for a problem does not exist. For instance, sitting at a computer for eight hours every day could eventually lead to lower back pain, muscle spasms, or wrist problems. It's better to catch the condition early than to wait until you are in great pain."

Cautions

Chiropractors should be particularly careful when it comes to elderly patients who have brittle bones. While pregnant women should be cautious about many medical treatments, a special table facilitates their chiropractic treatment. "Chiropractic therapy helps pregnant women with lower back pain—the realignment of the spine relieves the pressure," Dr. Davis explains. In certain cases "you can also realign the pelvis, which will make delivery a lot easier."

Choosing a Therapist

Chiropractic has a reputation as a back and neck cracking treatment. But fear of chiropractors is unjustified, Dr. Robinson says. "The adjustment procedures are virtually painless and complications are rare."

By and large, the number one question people should have answered when choosing a chiropractor should concern training. Because chiropractors are regulated in every state, you can contact chiropractic boards to find out if a particular chiropractor is licensed to practice.

Referrals from family and friends are a good way to be sure the practitioner you find is qualified to serve your needs. Any questions you have about chiropractic therapy and the experience, such as "Will it hurt?" "How many sessions does it usually take to address a particular problem?" and "Do you use any other alternative therapies?" should be asked prior to any manipulation so that you will know what to expect and feel more comfortable.

Cost

For an initial visit, an average cost ranges from $45 to $60 with follow-up visits for as little as $18 in some cases, depending on whether the visit is for preventive services or to treat an acute or chronic condition. More and more insurance plans are beginning to pay for visits to a chiropractor, especially when referred by a medical doctor. Check your plan to be sure.

"Chiropractic care is cheaper than back surgery," Dr. Robinson says. "And research shows that chiropractic treatment is more effective in treatment of lower back pain than any other care."

For example, for a patient with pain from an injured spinal disk, physicians often recommend that the disk be removed. But chiropractors typically demonstrate exercises, resting positions, and sitting positions that can alleviate the problem over a three- or four-month span by preventing the disk from being compressed. To determine just how serious a disk problem might be, Dr. Hudson performs an ultrasound test and then gives adjustments. "Now, if you have a disk that has popped altogether, you can't wait three or four months, you need immediate surgery. But if it's less severe, doing the therapy is a lot cheaper than paying a neurosurgeon, anesthesiologist, and the cost of a hospital stay."

Can I Do it Myself?

Chiropractors typically give patients therapeutic exercises to do at home, depending on the condition, but chiropractic adjustments should be performed only by a trained doctor.

For More Information

The American Black Chiropractic Association
1918 E. Grand Blvd.
St. Louis, MO 63107
314-531-0615

The American Chiropractic Association
1701 Clarendon Blvd.
Arlington, VA 22209
800-986-4636
703-276-8800

Chiropractic Care: Suggestions and Recommendations for At-home Care

If you are experiencing any kind of musculoskeletal discomfort, you may want to consider chiropractic care and treatment. The entire premise of chiropractic care is to move the patient from a "passive phase in their treatment to an active one as soon as possible," according to Dr. Jerome McAndrews, spokesperson for the American Chiropractic Association. After having manipulations performed, patients may be asked to take a walk around the block, or attempt to get into or out of a car without assistance. "Our goal is to restore mobility to the disfunctioning and immoble joints as well as the source of the original problem and the compensation points," said Dr. McAndrews. "Our body is designed like a swinging mobile. If one portion of the mobile is cut off or becomes imbalanced, the entire mobile will shift to accommodate that imbalance. The same is true for our bodies."

Chiropractors often recommend home self-care for patients as part of the active phase in health care. As part of chiropractic care that generally considers the "whole" patient, lifestyle factors such as diet, exercise, posture, and exercise are considered. Dr. Coralee Van Egmond of the International Chiropractic Association advises patients that as a part of home care you may be given one or more of the following recommended self-treatments.

ICE VERSUS HEAT

Often used for acute and chronic conditions, a patient may be instructed to use a combination of ice and heat or one or the other. Ice is often used for acute conditions and heat for chronic conditions like muscle aches. There are usually time limits on the use of both; for instance, a patient may be instructed to apply the remedy in increments of twenty minutes.

REST VERSUS EXERCISE

Oftentimes, bedrest is prescribed for severe chiropractic cases. It is believed, however, that prolonged periods of rest can actually do more harm than good. For example, only four days of bed rest can contribute to permanent muscle damage. If rest is recommended, it is usually in increments, or doctors will instruct patients to rest in supported positions. One common position is lying on the back with a pillow under the knees to provide support, or a roll under the neck to relieve pressure on the disks in the back, to support the natural curves of the spine and to rest muscles. Chiropractors often, when a patient is able, prescribe light exercises or walking, as a preferred treatment to complete rest.

STRETCHING

Stretching allows for the strengthening and stabilizing of the body and its various parts. Often, when prescribed by chiropractors, the goal is to provide increased flexibility. Specific stretching exercises can be tailored to a patient's needs and flexibility.

Colon Hydrotherapy

T. J. Vickers, a twenty-nine-year-old Washington, D.C., genealogist, was looking for an answer to her chronic constipation, lack of energy, and poor concentration. She consulted Dr. Andrea Sullivan, a naturopath and homeopath, who suggested a detoxification diet and colon hydrotherapy treatments. Vickers switched to a diet rich in fruits, vegetables, and fiber, then had three colonics in ten days. The combination of nutritious food, fasting, and several more colonics over the next ten days brought her immense relief. Vickers now says she is no longer constipated, has more energy than ever before, and is much better able to concentrate. Friends tell her that her skin has a healthier glow. Vickers sticks to the healthy diet, and says she doesn't feel as uptight or stressed as she used to. "The colonics have alleviated that backed-up feeling that I had. I've increased my activities tenfold and I can handle it, even with less sleep."

Vickers says she would recommend colon hydrotherapy to anyone. "There's nothing like walking out of there after having a colonic. I feel charged, I feel like floating, I feel relieved, released, like I can do anything."

Dr. Paul Brown Bodhise, a Philadelphia, Pennsylvania-based

African American chiropractor, naturopath, and herbalist, believes colon hydrotherapy "is very important for our people. I know it's highly underestimated in its ability to prevent some very serious maladies that affect our community."

What is Colon Hydrotherapy?

The colon is a hollow, muscular, tubelike organ that moves digested food from the small intestine to the rectum. While the colon reabsorbs water, nutrients, proteins, and cell salts from the food and returns it to the bloodstream, it is more broadly known for its role in waste disposal.

Waste material not eliminated through the colon, liver, kidneys, perspiration, or lungs can be stored in body tissue. Thus, congested bowels can contribute to problems ranging from abdominal discomfort to high blood pressure, allergies, menstrual problems, psoriasis, muscle weakness and severe fatigue, swollen legs, indigestion, asthma, backache, arthritis, and loss of memory or concentration. Many physicians believe that colon cancer is linked to the accumulation of waste that becomes toxic and causes the body to function less efficiently. "The buildup of fecal and waste material in the colon and the habit of holding bowel movements has caused many illnesses that affect the African American community," says Dr. Bodhise.

Colon hydrotherapy, sometimes called colon irrigation or colonic, is similar to a deep enema. While enemas release water about 6 to 12 inches into the digestive tract to clean the lower part of the colon (large intestine), the water in a colonic reaches the entire length of the colon, providing thorough cleansing.

Colon hydrotherapy also soothes and tones the colon, thereby helping it to function more efficiently. This reduces the burden on other organs and the lymphatic system, which protects the body from harmful bacteria. Colon hydrotherapy also exercises and strengthens the colon, enabling it to function more efficiently over the long run. As the colon fills with water, the colon muscles must contract in a wavelike motion to expel the liquid and waste. This movement strengthens the colon.

Overall, a cleansed colon is believed to improve the functions of the entire body. Those who have had the therapy often report a lighter, more energized feeling along with clearer skin and eyes, better elimination, improved posture, relief from gas, and a general feeling of improved health. Colon hydrotherapy benefits even people who aren't constipated, Dr. Bodhise says. "I think that periodic cleansing of the colon, every six months or so, is very important." In addition to prescribing colonics to some 70 percent of his patients, Dr. Bodhise says he has them himself whenever he starts feeling sluggish.

Some believe colon hydrotherapy dates to ancient Egypt. Like many natural-healing methods, it is regaining popularity today. Advances in sanitation and safety along with greater knowledge of proper techniques have made colon hydrotherapy more effective and less risky than in past years.

How Does it Work?

During colon hydrotherapy, water entering the colon softens the stools, so they can pass easily from the body. Practitioners believe that this cleansing of accumulated waste and toxins reduces the risk of diverticulitis (inflammation of tissue in the wall of the colon) and colon cancer.

The therapy is usually administered by a naturopathic doctor or trained colon hydrotherapist. In state-of-the-art practices, a small disposable tube about the size of a pencil is inserted (by the patient) into the rectum, allowing water to flow into the rectum and colon. Alternatively, a disposable speculum—a tube about five inches long and three quarters of an inch in diameter—is used. A water tube and a larger waste tube attach to the speculum.

A gentle infusion of warm, filtered water flows into and out of the body to remove accumulated fecal matter. An experienced, certified colon hydrotherapist knows how to work the body's meridians and pressure points and teach proper breathing techniques to minimize discomfort and maximize results from the therapy. The procedure may be repeated several times during a session.

The pressure from "bearing down" that occurs with enemas does not take place with colon hydrotherapy. The client rests comfortably on a table in a private room and elimination occurs during the session with no need to jump up and run to the bathroom. Little or no odor is apparent because waste exits the body through a sealed, clear tube. Clients are partially clothed during the treatment, which typically takes sixty to ninety minutes.

Best Uses
Colon hydrotherapy is commonly used for digestive disorders such as constipation, indigestion, and flatulence as well as backaches and fatigue. It relieves signs of a toxic colon, which include coated (abnormally colored) tongue, bad breath, sallow complexion, abnormal body odor, dark circles under the eyes, cold hands and feet, brittle nails and hair, sagging posture or pot belly, tension, allergies, indigestion, chronic headaches, irritability, nervousness, nausea, depression, and asthma. Some doctors recommend a full series of colon hydrotherapy as preparation for bowel surgery, because it can provide a more optimal surgical field and can potentially reduce the risk of postoperative complications by lessening bacteria at the suture site.

Cautions
Colon hydrotherapy is no panacea; it is most beneficial when combined with good nutrition, adequate fluids, and regular exercise.

William T. Tiller, N.D., president of the International Association for Colon Hydrotherapy (I-ACT), explains that some clients who take stimulants such as coffee, tea, and chocolate experience headaches and sometimes mild depression after colon hydrotherapy.

I-ACT recommends equipment approved by the Food and Drug Administration (FDA). Such devices feature temperature-controlled water, backflow prevention valves, pressure and temperature sensors, and a built-in chemical sanitizing unit or water purification unit. I-ACT provides lists of FDA-approved manufacturers. Therapists should use sterile-disposable rectal tubes or speculums. Those who use stainless-steel equipment should clean them with an autoclave machine, which kills germs with high heat.

Improperly administered colon hydrotherapy using non-FDA cleared equipment does have the potential to perforate the colon, a medical emergency that can release large amounts of toxins into the system at one time. FDA-cleared equipment maintains a lower pressure, to avoid perforation. I-ACT recommends that therapists allow the client to insert the rectal nozzle themselves.

Persons with heart trouble, severe hemorrhoids, colitis, or diverticulitis should not have colon hydrotherapy. Pregnant women should have the procedure only under the direction of a physician.

Finding a Therapist

Many naturopathic physicians, chiropractors and other alternative healers provide colon hydrotherapy. I-ACT certifies hydrotherapists who complete 100 hours of training at the beginning level and 500 hours of training at the intermediate level. When seeking a colon hydrotherapist, be sure to ask:

- whether the therapist is I-ACT certified

- whether their equipment is from an FDA-approved manufacturer

- whether the therapist will provide you with a new, sterile disposable speculum and rectal tube

- what you should eat and drink before and after a treatment

Cost

The cost of a treatment session usually ranges from $30 to $100. Most hydrotherapists recommend a series of twelve one-hour sessions to fully dislodge encrusted fecal matter; two the first week, two the second week, then weekly until the series is completed. Many clients then return every few months for maintenance.

Little research exists on the benefits of colon hydrotherapy, which is one reason insurance companies are reluctant to pay for it.

For More Information

International Association for Colon Hydrotherapy
P.O. Box 461285
San Antonio, TX 78246–1285
210–366–2888

A Healthy Colon and You

Are you feeling irritable and sluggish? Do you suffer from acne, cold hands and feet, depression, gas, or headaches? How about hypertension, allergies, asthma, or arthritis? If you answered yes to any of these ailments, the problem could be your colon. If your colon is not functioning properly or is even slightly blocked you could suffer from a wide range of health problems not commonly associated with the colon. How so? When the colon is congested and blocked, stagnant waste and toxins back up into the system and pollute the body. This process is called autointoxication, or "self-poisoning." Autointoxication causes blood poisoning that in turn causes disease. Improper elimination causes waste matter to build along the walls and pockets of the colon. Even a slight case of constipation can leave residue behind in the colon—sometimes for years. What's more, hardened fecal matter deposits can build up as thick as three inches and as hard as tire rubber. Inefficient bowel function can lead to nutrition deficiencies and prevent the body from absorbing minerals and nutrients through intestinal walls. Wide use and abuse of the over-the-counter laxatives mean many people, an estimated 70 million, will suffer from one of many colon-related disorders: colitis, ileitis, diverticulitis, constipation, or worse, may be one of the 100,000 who have a colostomy, a surgical procedure that creates an excretory opening for the colon, each year. What's the good news in all of this? Well, a properly maintained colon can mean the dissipation of many ailments. A colonic cleansing can remove hardened waste and promote healthy digestive function once again. A lighter more energetic feeling can be the result of proper colon maintenance.

Herbal Remedies

When Paul Bodhise, D.C., says, "You are responsible for your own life," he speaks from firsthand experience. In the early 1970s, Dr. Bodhise returned home to Philadelphia, Pennsylvania, from Vietnam with mysterious lumps, bumps, and sores on his face. The puzzling illness sent him to the hospital, where the combat veteran received a shocking wake-up call. The physician who examined him was also working on another patient who had just arrived with a gunshot wound. "He came out from another room with bloody hands and touched my face to examine the bumps," Dr. Bodhise recalls. "He looked at me and said he didn't know what it was, and he asked me if I knew. Then he walked out of the room. I left that hospital with two handprints of someone else's

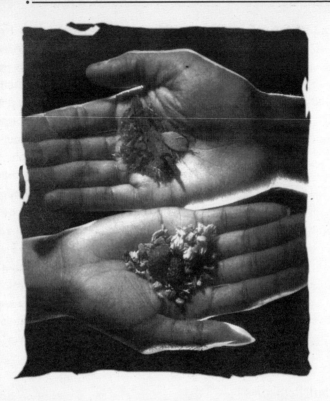

blood on my face." That's when he knew he had to take his health into his own hands.

The first step was finding the resources. Dr. Bodhise discovered an Islamic group whose members handed out information about herbs, suggesting that African Americans refrain from eating meat, sugar, and dairy products. He accepted their suggestions, although it wasn't easy. "Back then (the early 1970s) they called me a health food nut," Dr. Bodhise says in reference to his friends and relatives who didn't understand his choice to pursue natural healing. "I said to myself that if I can just keep myself healthy and beautiful, then people will see the effects of the herbs and better understand my choices and perhaps incorporate some of them into their own lives. All it takes is a seeking mind and spirit."

And about those lumps and bumps? "One day I realized that I hadn't noticed them for a long time," says Dr. Bodhise, who went on to earn his Doctor of Naturopathy degree and to become licensed in chiropractic. "I have been fine ever since." Dr. Bodhise says his willingness to do the work led him to healing. "I'm convinced that in herbal healing, there is a solution to every disease if folks would just commit to doing the work to find it."

What are Herbal Remedies?

Herbalism is the study of the medicinal qualities of plants and naturally produced products (such as honey). Since ancient times, herbs have been used by virtually every culture to relieve pain, discomfort, and disease. It was ancient Africans—the Egyptians— who as far back as 3000 B.C. began cataloguing herbs according to their effects. Based on these and countless other such descriptions of herbs and their effects, contemporary naturopathic physicians and herbalists know how to treat a variety of ailments. "Naturopathic physicians are trained to match the action of the herb with the action of the body," explains Andrea Sullivan, N.D., a Washington, D.C.-based naturopath.

Plant-based therapies are far older than the prescription drugs that in the last century have come to dominate the medical field. While many prescription drugs contain plant ingredients, they also contain synthetic chemicals made to mimic the action and effectiveness of certain herbs. Some believe that prescription drugs, which can have toxic side effects, can do more harm than good, throwing out of balance a body that needs to regain its equilibrium.

"Prescription drugs are designed to kill a diseased cell and stop it from producing," Dr. Bodhise explains. "The mentality is that if you kill the cell that is out of control, you can save the person. Herbology, however, uses herbs to strengthen the immune system so that the body can heal itself."

"We use herbs all the time," begins New York-based Courtney

Witherspoon, O.M.D., who specializes in acupuncture and herbal healing. "We live off of plants that nourish us and give us minerals that feed our bones, teeth and eyes. Herbology is nothing new, but we have come to use certain plants for everyday foods and seasonings and others for medicinal purposes."

How Do They Work?

Herbs support the body and help it to operate optimally. Herbs can help when allopathic medicine fails to get to the root of a health condition. Dr. Witherspoon recalls a patient who experienced pains and cramping in her legs as an adverse reaction to a hepatitis vaccine. Her physicians gave her muscle relaxants, but they were ineffective; eventually the woman was unable to walk. Dr. Witherspoon, determining that the vaccine had injured the patient's liver—the body's blood purifier—prescribed a tea of dandelion, red clover, and nettle. "Dandelion supports the liver; red clover clears the blood; the nettle supports the blood system," Dr. Witherspoon explains. After only two days, the woman could stand once again. "Herbs can change the physiology of the body so that the body can produce its own medicine," Dr. Bodhise adds.

Like many practitioners, Dr. Witherspoon offered her patient specific preparation instructions. "I told her to boil the dandelion root for ten minutes in a covered pot, and then pour it over the red clover and nettle leaves in a cup, cover for ten minutes and then strain it. In general, you have to boil herbs when they are in the root or seed form. You don't boil leaves but rather you pour boiling water over them, strain them out, and then drink the tea." Such preparation provides the maximum effects of the herbs. "Some people prefer tinctures [little bottles of the herb in liquid form], but someone in a crisis needs to make a tea," she adds. "Celestial Seasonings or any other kind already in a tea bag is not strong enough. You need the tea directly from the herb itself to make a difference in a condition. Pills are okay, but it has been my experience that the teas are most effective."

Because liquids are fast-acting, Dr. Sullivan also prefers them over pills, although pills hide the bitter taste of many of the herbs. "The bitter taste is a part of the medicinal action," Dr. Sullivan says. "If you add sugar you'll end up with something like the ineffective cough syrups on the market."

Dr. Bodhise recommends drinking teas throughout the day when trying to heal a particular condition. "You also have to drink lots of water (eight to twelve 8-ounce glasses a day) to help flush the body of toxins as the herbs jump-start the immune system."

Best Uses

Herbal remedies are useful for a variety of ailments, from colds and allergies to indigestion, bronchitis, asthma, arthritis, and cancer. Saw palmetto helps treat diabetes and prostate cancer; catnip helps to reduce pain; *Aloe vera* relieves burns. Echinacea, goldenseal, osha root, poke root, and other antibacterial and antiviral herbs stimulate the immune system to fight off a cold. Horehound, aspidosperma, and cabbage soothe the bronchial passages and help to clear mucus; poke root and echinacea are good for sore throats.

Herbs have certain affinities for particular organs. "For example, fenugreek and elderberry have affinities for the lungs," Dr. Witherspoon explains. "Fennel has an affinity for the digestive tract. General herbs like echinacea and goldenseal act throughout the body."

Cautions

Herbs can be powerful. Some, such as goldenseal, foxglove, and licorice root, can be toxic if taken in large doses; ginseng and licorice root can increase blood pressure. The popular herb goldenseal, which jump-starts the immune system, has important antibiotic properties, especially when combined with echinacea. But it can also lower blood sugar or cause nervousness. "Goldenseal should not be taken every day, but only on an as-needed basis," Dr. Witherspoon says. Fennel in large amounts can cause diarrhea.

Americans sometimes incorrectly take Chinese herbs individually; they are designed to be taken in combination. "Taken by themselves, some of these herbs can cause rectal bleeding or blood clots," Dr. Witherspoon says. "Dong quai is being used more and more by itself for female problems, but this is not advisable." She also warns against taking ginseng alone, which in excess can cause nervous restlessness. "If you are treating something for up to six months and it has not gone away, you should see a doctor—a naturopathic physician, preferably," Dr. Sullivan believes. "Taking herbs without any guidance or knowledge of what you are doing can be one of the biggest threats to your health. A qualified practitioner can help you take the right herbs in the proper amount."

Choosing a Therapist

Some people take weekend courses on herbs and call themselves herbalists. Find out where a practitioner was trained and who trained them. Is it a mail-order school or does the school have a real campus? "I don't believe you can treat the human body unless you have seen one," Dr. Sullivan says. "Naturopathic physicians must know everything a medical doctor knows, like the physiology and biochemistry of the body. You dissect a cadaver to learn how everything works together." Someone who hasn't gone through this kind of training can do more harm than good. "You wouldn't go to any other doctor who wasn't accredited," Dr. Sullivan says. "So why settle for less in a natural doctor?" Three schools in the United States offer the Doctor of Naturopathy degree: Bastyr University in Seattle, Washington; National College of Naturopathic Medicine in Portland, Oregon; and College of Naturopathic Medicine and Health Sciences in Scottsdale, Arizona. Contact the American Association of Naturopathic Physicians (see end of chapter) for a referral to a therapist in your area.

Watch a therapist to ensure you are getting someone who practices what they preach. "Does the person have a glowing face, a happy demeanor? Is the office pleasant and clean?" Dr. Bodhise asks. And be sure to ask whether a therapist works with other practitioners, such as acupuncturists. "Avoid a therapist who suggests that only his or her approach to your problem will work," Dr. Bodhise advises. "There are hundreds of herbs and different approaches to using them. My attitude has always been: 'I am only one ray of the sun'."

In addition, find someone who has a thorough understanding of how herbs work in the body. For instance, some who study herbology in a weekend course memorize specific herbs to use for various ailments without actually studying herbs to know what might be best for a particular person with a specific ailment. In addition to the eyes, Dr. Witherspoon also examines the tongue, nails, quality of skin; she takes the pulse and palpates the stomach. "You want a practitioner who can give you a thorough exam and then have a full knowledge of herbs that can help you," she says.

Cost

When it comes to comparing the cost of mainstream and herbal treatments, it's easy to find yourself in a Catch-22. On the one hand, herbs are inexpensive compared with prescription and over-the-counter medicine. On the other, naturopathic doctors are not usually covered by insurance policies. Insurance companies will pay for you to see a medical doctor—but will that fix what ails you? You may find that the best approach is to visit a physician when it is appropriate to do so, but don't stay away from herbalists—even if you have to foot the bill yourself.

Herbs purchased from a health food store in bulk are the least expensive. If you buy the herbs in pill form (which are still less costly than most prescription drugs), find out how quickly the store changes its stock. Opt for the freshest product available. Instead of buying pills off the shelf, you can also have the store grind down the bulk herbs, then buy your own capsules and make your own pills. This helps ensure that the herbs are fresh and haven't sat on the shelf for a long time.

Can I Do it Myself?

Anyone who eats well, exercises, drinks fresh juices, and eats green leafy vegetables and sea vegetables already practices herbal healing. For more information, read books about herbs, then discuss your questions with a skilled healer. Remember, the treatment of long-term or serious disorders should be left to professionals.

For More Information

American Association of Naturopathic Physicians
601 Valley St., Suite 105
Seattle, WA 98109–4229
206–323–7610; (206) 298–0126; Fax (206) 298–0129

American Naturopathic Medical Association
P.O. Box 19221
Las Vegas, NV 89132
702–796–9067

Finding and Using Herbal Remedies to Treat Common Ailments

Herbs can be used to treat a variety of conditions and ailments from disorders of the skin, digestive, respiratory and reproductive systems. Herbs also provide relief from symptoms like headaches, PMS, help alleviate chemotherapy symptoms and many many more. If you believe that an herbal remedy can provide benefit to an ailment, it is best to consult an herbalist or a physician who advocates the use of herbs. Once under supervision you may want to start making your own remedies at home and you will need to find a source of good, healthy herbs to get started. First, large, well-stocked health food stores carry a wide variety of herbs. They can also be found in large organic health markets or grocery stores. Mail order is also a common location for herbs. Herbs purchased in stores will display the exact name, i.e., chamomile, on the packaging and will list and describe its other ingredients. As with food and other types of products, the manufacturing process affects the strength and healing value of herbs. Consumers should inspect packaging on herbs and should understand how they were processed. Avoid older looking herbs that have been on the shelf for some time. Herbs should also be stored in a glass or ceramic container in a cool, dark place. Once purchased, herbs should be used within one year of purchase because they often lose their effectiveness over time.

When preparing herbal remedies keep in mind that the typical ratio of medicinal doses is 1 ounce of dried herbs or 2 ounces of fresh herbs to 2 cups of water. Usually the herbs will absorb half of the water used in making a remedy. For remedies taken by mouth you may find the solution extremely bitter and unpalatable. Try adding honey to make the solution more edible.

Here is a list of some common mixtures of herbs easily prepared in the home:

Tea or Infusion: Herbs are placed into a teapot and boiling water is added to make into a drinkable solution. Once boiled, the solution should be allowed to sit for fifteen minutes. Strain before drinking.

Tincture: This remedy uses alcohol instead of water to release the active ingredient in the herb. Using vodka (never rubbing alcohol), add enough to cover the herb in a glass or ceramic container. Seal and let stand for about two weeks, storing in a cool, dark place. Mixture should be shaken twice daily. Once fermented, mix with juice to disguise bitter taste.

Syrup: Used mostly to disguise bitter-tasting herbs. Herbs are first prepared as an infusion or decoction (see below). Strain the mixture in a small saucepan using low heat. Once strained, stir in honey—about 2 tablespoons or according to taste.

Decoction: Is made by boiling dried roots or woody parts of herbs like bark in water. Once boiled, herbs should be placed into a saucepan and cold water can be added. Bring to a boil again, simmering gently for about an hour and until the volume has been reduced slightly (about a third). Strain before using.

Compresses: To be used for skin problems and sore muscles and joints. To make, take a small towel or washcloth and soak in hot herbal tea. Wring out and place on affected area. Cover soaked towel on skin with a dry towel to keep heat in place. Repeat as needed.

Homeopathy

Andrea Sullivan was thirty years old and she had it all: a doctorate in sociology, an impressive career, an expensive car. But she was also exhausted, overweight, and full of acne. Despite her material comforts, she felt dispirited and emotionally disconnected. A friend referred Sullivan to a naturopathic doctor who helped her identify the racism she'd experienced as a root cause of her unwellness.

As she healed, Sullivan decided to become a naturopath and

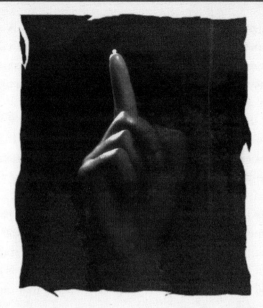

bring this medicine to other African Americans. After studying chemistry, physiology, anatomy, biology, and psychology at Howard University, she enrolled at Bastyr University in Seattle, one of the nation's three schools of naturopathy, where she learned counseling, nutrition, herbal medicine, acupuncture, and homeopathy.

Today Sullivan enjoys a thriving homeopathic and naturopathic practice in Washington, D.C., where her office has a three-month waiting list for new patients. Her patients speak enthusiastically of how she has changed their lives for the better. Walter House III, fifty-two years old, of Columbus, Ohio, says Dr. Sullivan has helped him lose weight, get in shape, lower his blood pressure, and improve his memory and concentration. Washington, D.C., resident Eleanor Thompson, also fifty-two, credits Dr. Sullivan for helping her stay healthy and cancer-free after a 1991 mastectomy. Thompson had been seeing Sullivan for two years when she was given her first homeopathic remedy to help her deal with work-related stress. "I felt better in a day or two, and haven't craved crunchy foods, as I did before taking the remedy."

Dr. Sullivan, a founding member of the American Association of Naturopathic Physicians and board member of the National Center for Homeopathy, often speaks to church and civic groups in the Washington, D.C., area. "As Black Americans approach the twenty-first century, we need to take responsibility for healing ourselves," she writes in her book, *A Path to Healing: A Guide to Wellness for Body, Mind and Soul* (Doubleday, 1998). "I think the depth of our suffering mentally, emotionally, spiritually and physically can be approached and affected by homeopathy in ways that conventional medicine cannot touch," says Dr. Sullivan. "Homeopathic remedies create freedom from limitations, whether those limits are mental, emotional, spiritual, or physical. If you are preoccupied with depression or arthritis, you can't live your life in the way that spirit intended. The depth of our suffering is dramatic and we need treatment that is equally as dramatic, that can change the energy of who we are."

What is Homeopathy?

Homeopathy was founded by Samuel Hahnemann, a German doctor, in 1790. Seeking a way to effectively treat malaria, he took a dose of Peruvian bark (quinine), which was widely prescribed for the disease. Hahnemann promptly developed malaria. When he stopped taking the bitter medicine, the symptoms disappeared. Intrigued, Hahnemann tested hundreds of animal, mineral, and vegetable substances on himself and colleagues. Every test supported the idea that a substance that induces symptoms in a healthy person can relieve the same symptoms in a sick person. Hahnemann named his discovery homeopathy based on the Greek words *homoion* ("similar") and *pathein* ("disease" or "suffering").

Homeopathy is based on Hahnemann's Law of Similars: like cures like. For example, a remedy that causes fever and headache in a well person will relieve someone who is sick with the same type of fever and headache. Well-known conventional medicines based on the Law of Similars include vaccines, allergy treatments, and the heart medicine nitroglycerine.

Homeopathy uses small doses of natural animal, mineral, or vegetable substances to help the body heal itself. While other forms of medicine target the causes of disease (viruses, bacteria, etc.), homeopathic remedies treat specific symptoms on an individual basis. Two persons suffering from the same ailment may have very different symptoms, and therefore, need different remedies. The key to healing is to find the remedy that most closely matches the patient's physical, mental, and emotional symptoms. The remedy acts as a catalyst to restore good health.

While some homeopathic remedies, such as chamomile and marigold, evoke positive images, mercury and arsenic are part of homeopathic care as well. Even the deadliest poisons are safe in homeopathic form because they are so highly diluted that little of the original substance remains. The substance is mixed in alcohol to obtain an extract known as a tincture, which is mixed with more alcohol and vigorously shaken. Small sugar pills are saturated with the liquid dilution to become homeopathic remedies. A few of the remedies are placed under the patient's tongue where they are absorbed into the bloodstream. Some homeopathic remedies are available as gels and salves for external use.

Homeopathy came to the United States in 1832. By the turn of the century practitioners had established twenty-two homeopathic medical schools, 100 homeopathic hospitals, and more than 1,000 homeopathic pharmacies. "Because abolitionists William Lloyd Garrison and Zabina Eastman were strong proponents of homeopathy, and also because many individual homeopaths were politically progressive, homeopathy became identified with causes of female and black emancipation," adds Robert Ullman, N.D., and Judith Reichenberg Ullman, N.D., authors of *Homeopathy: Medicine for the 21st Century.*

Virtually since its inception in the United States, homeopathy has faced hostility from physicians who likened it to quackery. But as managed care complicates conventional medicine and patients grow increasingly frustrated by the cost and limitations of drug therapies, growing numbers of Americans are turning to homeopathy. Americans made an estimated 4.8 million visits to homeopathic practitioners in 1990 by one tally. The National Center for Homeopathy lists some 3,000 homeopathic practitioners, including about a dozen African Americans, in the United States.

Homeopathy is practiced widely throughout the world, including Germany (where it was discovered), India, Mexico, South America, Great Britain, Greece, Scandinavia, France, and the former Soviet Union. On the African continent, homeopathy is practiced in South Africa, Egypt, and Morocco, according to Dr. Sullivan and Dana Ullman, M.P.H., director of Homeopathic Educational Services. African American enthusiasts of homeopathy include Dizzy Gillespie, Tina Turner, Camille Cosby, and Whoopi Goldberg.

How Does it Work?

In classic homeopathy, a practitioner prescribes a single remedy based on a patient's physical, mental, and emotional health. This is called constitutional prescribing and is commonly used for chronic health problems.

A homeopathic doctor is needed for constitutional prescribing. Constitutional homeopathic treatment begins with an in-depth patient interview during which the doctor learns enough about the patient's physical, mental, and emotional health history, symptoms, habits, and traits to select the most appropriate remedy. It is common for the doctor to inquire about family health patterns, childhood illnesses, sleep patterns, sexual desires, food cravings and aversions, strong likes and dislikes, and how the patient likes to spend their time. The questions may strike you as absurd or irrelevant, but they can yield valuable information. For instance, a strong aversion to heat or cold might indicate one remedy; the tendency to sigh and cry easily might indicate another.

First-time patients are often shocked that a visit to a homeopath may include little or no physical examination. "It was very different, she didn't touch me," recalls Nevada Warren about her initial visit to Dr. Andrea Sullivan. "She just talked and asked a lot of questions. Most doctors ask about your symptoms and the health challenges that you're faced with. Dr. Sullivan asked general questions about me, my lifestyle, my eating, my dreaming—things that sounded very unusual to me." Because they are so intent on listening to a patient as well as closely observing the patient's tone of voice, body language, and overall demeanor, homeopaths may seem somewhat detached during a consultation.

When a practitioner cannot talk with a patient in person, it is not unusual to work by phone. By learning about symptoms and assessing the patient's anxiety, lethargy, or other emotional states through tone of voice, diagnosis and treatment can proceed. Of course it is preferred to have an in-person consultation.

Practitioners who determine that a condition cannot be treated by homeopathy alone may prescribe conventional medical treatment, then select homeopathic remedies to speed recovery and possibly reduce the undesirable side effects of drug treatment.

Best Uses

Homeopathy is useful for a variety of short-term and chronic health problems. About 80 percent of homeopathic patients are seen for chronic complaints, mainly asthma, depression, ear infections, allergies, headache/migraine, neurological disorders, allergy, dermatitis/eczema, arthritis, and high blood pressure, according to a 1992 survey of members of the American Institute of Homeopathy (AIH). Studies suggest that homeopathy is also effective in treating sore throat, cough and flu, PMS, menopause, menstrual cramps, morning sickness, bronchitis and hay fever, arthritis, digestive disorders, depression and anxiety, chronic fatigue syndrome, acute childhood diarrhea, colic and teething pain in infants, and sports and exercise injuries.

The remedies have virtually no adverse side effects.

Cautions

If your symptoms do not respond to homeopathic treatment over time, you may need conventional medicine. "If a disease is serious and destructive, or if there are good conventional treatments for the problem, withholding homeopathic therapy or reserving it for supportive therapy complementary to conventional medicine may be important to prevent harm by progression of the illness," write Wayne B. Jonas and Jennifer Jacobs in *Healing with Homeopathy: The Complete Guide.* Cancer often brings few symptoms, so homeopathy shouldn't be used as the primary treatment of this disease.

When disease involves major anatomical changes, such as hardening of the arteries, a broken leg, or a foreign body in the eye, homeopathy alone will usually not reverse them. The same holds true when chronic disease causes anatomical changes. Arthritis begins with many symptoms and few anatomical changes until it is quite advanced. Homeopathy relieves pain and inflammation in early stages of arthritis but will not restore deformed joint function in later stages.

Often only a single dose of a remedy is needed. Practitioners recommend taking the lowest possible dose for the least possible time. When you self-treat, it is important not to combine remedies or change from one to another too quickly. Otherwise, symptoms can become difficult to distinguish, or may even become more pronounced. When taking homeopathic remedies, whether they are constitutionally or self-prescribed, avoid the following, which can neutralize the remedies:

• Coffee, regular or decaffeinated.

- Camphor in any form, including products like Vicks Vaporub, Ben-Gay, Tiger Balm, Noxzema skin cream, and other cosmetics and personal hygiene products, including some nail polishes.

- Recreational drugs of all kinds.

- Conventional pharmaceutical medications (unless they are needed to treat a chronic problem such as hypertension or diabetes). With earaches, headaches, or the like, it is all right to take a dose of aspirin or acetaminophen for pain relief while the remedy is working.

- Electric blankets, which some homeopaths believe can potentially neutralize remedies.

- Dental work involving anesthesia.

- Mint, including candy and toothpaste.

Choosing a Therapist

Because homeopathy is not regulated, shop carefully for a practitioner. If you have a serious or chronic health problem, select a classic homeopath with plenty of experience who has completed a major professional training course in homeopathy, such as those offered by a leading homeopathic organization or school of naturopathy. The practitioner should include the results of tests and information from your medical records in any treatment. Organizations such as the National Center for Homeopathy (address on p. 155) can refer you to homeopaths, including African American practitioners.

Choose a practitioner who is knowledgeable and flexible enough to recognize both the advantages and limitations of homeopathy and to prescribe accordingly. Some questions to ask a practitioner:

- What kind of training and experience have you had? Do you consult with more experienced professional homeopaths about challenging cases?

- What kind of information will be covered in the consultation? Will you conduct a physical examination? What, if any, information do I need to provide?

- Do you supplement homeopathic therapy with suggestions for a healthier lifestyle, or with other alternative or conventional treatments?

- What are your office policies, fee structure? What insurance information do I need to know about?

Cost

The average first visit to a homeopathic physician lasts an hour and costs $137, according to a nationwide AIH member survey. The average follow-up visit lasts twenty-five minutes and costs $55. Most health insurers cover visits to homeopathic practitioners because they are licensed as medical doctors, doctors of osteopathy, etc.

Can I Treat Myself?

While it is best to see a homeopathic practitioner for serious or chronic health problems, many laypersons purchase the remedies, which are available over the counter, to self-treat minor ailments. Growing numbers of homeopathic pharmacies are appearing throughout the United States, and remedies are carried in virtually all natural food stores. National retail chains including CVS, Kmart, Eckerd, Drug Emporium, Meijers, Osco, Payless, Revco, Target, Thrifty, FredMeyer, and Walgreens carry homeopathic medicines, which average $3 to $7 per package.

For More Information
Homeopathic Academy of Naturopathic Physicians
12132 SE Foster Pl.
Portland, OR 97266
(503) 761–3298

National Center for Homeopathy
801 North Fairfax St.
Suite 306
Alexandria, VA 22314
(703) 548–7790

International Foundation for Homeopathy
P.O. Box 7
Edmonds, WA 98020
(206) 776–4147

For a "Healing With Homeopathy" self-care kit, call:
Arrowroot Standard Direct
1–800–234–8879

Boiron, USA
1–800–BOIRON–1

Homeopathic Educational Services
Berkeley, CA
1–800–359–9051

Common Homeopathic Remedies

Homeopathic remedies like many other remedies can be found in
health food stores, organic food markets, or by mail order. If you

are just beginning to explore the wonders of homeopathic care, it is advised that you consult with a homeopathic practitioner first. Ailments treated in the home should be minor, like cuts, scrapes, and burns—ailments that would normally not require medical intervention. For starters, you may want some of the following treatments in your home medicine cabinet:

Aconitum: Used for the beginning stages of minor illness like colds, chickenpox, measles and mumps, insomnia and earaches, toothaches and headaches.

Apis mellifica: Used to treat bee stings and other insect bites, sunburn, rashes, and splinter injuries.

Arnica: Essential in treating injuries due to falls, hits, and bruises. Also soothes emotional hurts.

Arsenicum album: Used to treat severe exhaustion, stomach and intestinal disorders, and shock.

Belladona: Treats fever and disorders with symptoms that include severe pulsating and pounding of the skin.

Bryona: Relieves irritability, stabbing irritating pain and physical weakness.

Cepa: Treats colds and problems with the ears, nose and throat.

Chamomilla: Used to treat extreme irritability and restlessness, overreacting, and low pain tolerance.

Gelsemium: Treats colds and fever characterized by tiredness, anxious weakness with tremors and dizziness.

Hamamelis: Is used to treat hemorrhoids and varicose veins. Can be used topically as a salve or internally.

Hypericum: Treats bruises and contusions on the nails and fingers. Is helpful after dental treatment, surgery and postpartum.

Ignatia: Effective in treating the aftermath of worries and sorrow and lovesickness.

Ledum: Is vital in treating injuries caused by nails, rakes, thorns, and insect bites. Also treats eye injuries, pulled liga-ments, and sprains.

Nux vomica: Is used to treat mental overstimulations and failure to perform. Also used after misuse of stimulants such as caffeine.

Phosphorus: Treats nervous overload and overstimulation.

Pulsatilla: Treats "clinginess" in children and extreme sensitivity in adults.

Sepia: Treats exhaustion, burnout, and anxiety. Empha-sizes treatment of the female organs.

While assembling your homeopathic "medicine cabinet," you may find many odd sounding names or even alpha-numeric references. These references—for instance, Sepia C1 or Corallium rubrum D6—are simply measuring formulas similar to those a pharmacist would use when measuring dosage amounts for patients. Dr. Samuel Hahnemann, while formalizing homeopathic treatments, created a system of measurements and recommended dosages; the process is called diluting. The most widely used measuring scale is the C scale or hundredth. In this measurement, one drop of the original solution is added to 100 drops of a carrier solution. So, if you have a prescription of Belladonna D6 (D equaling one-tenth or 1/10), this means 10 drops of the original solu-tion to 600 drops of a carrier solution.

Massage Therapy

Bonita Buchanan-Jones knew she had the touch from as early as ten years of age. "My Dad was a schoolteacher, and he had high blood pressure," she recalls. "He would come home from work and tell me to massage his neck and shoulders while he sat in his favorite chair. And like clockwork, every day, I would knock him

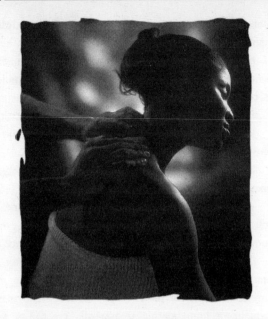

out. In no time at all, he had relaxed into a deep sleep. It was then that I knew I wanted to do something to help people."

To Buchanan-Jones, helping folks took on a variety of meanings. Her father had given her a love for reading, and because her mother was a nurse, there were always plenty of medical books and journals for her to devour. "Barely out of elementary school, I was reading medical journals and books every chance I got," she says. When she went to college, Buchanan-Jones had every intention of becoming a doctor. But after receiving her undergraduate degree, she decided that medical school was not for her. Tuition was a consideration; so was the time commitment. But what stopped her most of all, she admits, were physicians' attitudes. "Many doctors seem to think, 'The patient comes to me, and I cure him.' I was more interested in helping folks cure themselves," Buchanan-Jones says. From her experience with her father, she knew that if she could just get people to relax, their bodies would take over and do the rest.

Today, as a licensed massage therapist in Boston, Massachusetts, Buchanan-Jones has found that her soothing touch has helped her clients relax and heal. "When people want healing they will come to me, but they must first be willing to give up the tension inside their muscles and to give up what's inside their heads," she says.

What is Massage Therapy?

Anyone who's ever touched their own body to rub away a nagging pain or gently kneaded a loved one's aching back has an intuitive understanding of massage. "The difference between what we as trained therapists do and what you do as a loving friend is simply that we know where to rub and how much pressure to apply to bring about relief," says Connie Shanks, C.M.T., a Jackson, Mississippi, massage therapist.

By formal definition, massage is the therapeutic manipulation of the soft tissues of the body using strokes that include kneading (using fingers and thumbs to squeeze and roll the flesh), friction pressure (small circular movements), and tapping. These techniques help the therapist return your body to its most relaxed and healthful state. If you were a piece of dough, stress would make you a tight ball. The therapist's job, like a master chef, is to smooth you out. In a relaxed state, you are better prepared to deal with tension and stress and your body's defenses stay in top form. In addition, massage therapists sometimes apply heat or cold, or instruct a client about exercises they can do at home to prolong the benefits of your massage.

Since ancient times when Egyptians, Greeks, and Romans used massage as a way to jump-start the body into healing itself, massage has been used to relieve pain and discomfort by inducing a natural state of relaxation. In fact, massage was practiced in hospitals throughout the United States as a part of physical therapy until the 1950s when physical therapy became a separate discipline. When antibiotics were introduced as a virtual cure-all, during that same time period, people began to see modern medicine as the source for all their healing needs, and interest in massage declined.

When massage regained popularity in the 1970s, it was dominated by two distinct personalities. Massage represented either a luxury for rich White folks or a backroom pleasure in a seedy part of town. To African Americans, both images have given massage a bad name and kept many of us from understanding massage as a serious healing act. Michelle Spillman, C.M.T., an Atlanta, Georgia, massage therapist, believes lack of exposure has inhibited African Americans from taking advantage of the benefits of massage. "We know a lot about clothes, taking care of our hair and nails, but the idea of taking off your clothes in front of a stranger is just not appealing to us," she says. "So part of the job is educating people about what massage is."

"Most people don't know they can afford to get a massage," says Los Angeles, California-based massage therapist Louretta Walker, C.M.T. "Or they think, 'If I get an extra $45 in my pocket, I'm going to buy me something with it.' They think massage is a luxury and not something that is essential. But the brothers and sisters I work on, when they see the differences in their bodies after just one session, they know that a massage is something that they definitely need."

"Many of us [African Americans] don't know that massage is preventive medicine," Walker adds. "Massage connects you with who you really are. Many of us don't know the importance of having the body, mind and spirit working together—something massage promotes. When you have all three working simultaneously, you can accomplish just about anything."

The most common type of massage in the United States is Swedish massage. Per Heinrik Ling (1776–1839) is credited with systematizing the modern western practice of massage in the early 1800s. Ling suffered with rheumatism and found relief through massage. He integrated emerging knowledge of anatomy, physiology, and circulation of the blood with traditional eastern healing techniques and his own set of physical exercises to develop Swedish massage.

In the United States, Swedish massage is the most popular, although many massage therapists use a combination of Swedish, sports, and deep-tissue massage. "A Swedish massage is like a circulatory relaxation massage that gets the blood flowing and helps the client feel warm and relaxed. The strokes are not too deep," Spillman says. "With a sports massage, you go a little deeper because you are trying to flush the muscles of toxins like lactic acid that build up after a workout. Stretching exercises may also be involved. Deep-tissue massage is more about the structure of a person. You go deeper into the tissue layers to get the circulation flowing back into the muscles."

Other types of massage include Rolfing, therapeutic massage, and shiatsu (also considered a form of acupressure). Rolfing relies primarily on deep massage of the muscles and connective tissues. Named for its founder, American biochemist Dr. Ida Rolf, Rolfing theorizes that when we are aligned, gravity flows through us, allowing us to move more easily. The therapist aims to realign the body structure, restoring balance. Therapeutic massage consists mainly of soothing strokes and rubbing. It is especially useful for the relief of pain or physical discomfort. It speeds recovery after a heart attack and eases the suffering of cancer patients. Shiatsu is an ancient form of pressure-point massage based on the principles of acupuncture. Instead of using needles, pressure is applied to key points that relieve ailments such as stress, headaches, fever, and pain.

How Does it Work?

Getting a massage can be intimidating for some. Trust between a client and a therapist is the first step toward increased comfort. "I find there is an unwillingness on the part of many African Americans to let people get close to them," Buchanan-Jones says. "To get the most out of a massage session, you must be willing to trust the therapist and let him or her guide you in the healing process."

Before a massage session begins, reputable therapists start by having new clients fill out an intake form. "The intake form asks questions about medical history and also asks the client to explain why he or she is getting a massage," Shanks says. First-time clients may not know what type of massage they need. The intake form helps the therapist know what type of massage will be best. "Before a session, I will ask, 'What do you want in this session?' and most of the time I'll get an answer like, 'I just want to relax because I've been under a lot of stress,' so I'll do a calming Swedish massage," Buchanan-Jones says. 'If they say, 'I've been in a car accident so I have a stiff neck,' I won't go too deep, and in our initial conversation over the phone, I will advise a person to use ice or heat on their troubled spots before they come."

While you can receive a massage fully dressed, most therapists ask clients to remove their clothes and jewelry for maximum benefit. "If clients are uncomfortable fully undressing, they can keep their underwear on," Spillman says. Therapists generally cover their clients with a sheet or towel. During the massage, only the body part being worked on is uncovered.

Walker usually begins a session by trepidating a client (holding a body part and shaking it), who lies facedown. "Trepidating allows the body to become very fluid," she says. "It makes hard and tight tissues melt, relaxing you into another place."

After trepidating, a therapist begins working on individual parts or sections of the body, usually beginning from the neck and shoulders and working all the way down to the toes. Most therapists work toward the heart, which is said to keep the blood flowing in the proper direction.

Depending on how long your session is, the therapist may then ask you to turn over, still fully covered, and begin massaging the front of your body, perhaps beginning from the feet and legs and working up to the neck and head. Private areas remain covered at all times.

If a therapist massages an area that contains pent-up stress or tension, many clients experience emotional release. "A background in psychology can help a therapist be better prepared to deal with people's issues that may arise during a massage," Walker says. "Touching the right place may make a client recall an earlier painful experience that is recorded in the body in that place. This could result in a client crying or showing other emotions."

"Emotional releases are not why most people come. They come to relax, but what they find is that relaxing releases a lot of issues that have been inside for a long time," Shanks says. While some African Americans may not be comfortable with the idea of having their emotions out on the table in front of a stranger, therapists say the full benefits of massage can be realized only through a willingness to surrender. "Get the issues out of the tissues!" Shanks advises.

Best Uses

With African Americans suffering in large numbers from chronic diseases such as hypertension, high blood pressure, and heart disease, stress control is all-important. "Half of my clientele has high blood pressure," Spillman says. "Getting a massage relaxes your nervous system and helps lower blood pressure."

While bones give a person structure (making us solid), muscles help hold the bones in place. Tight, tensed, and stressed muscles impede blood circulation. "Blood carries oxygen throughout the body, but it also helps dispose of carbon dioxide and toxins," Spillman says. "If circulation is blocked, blood does not flow properly and toxins build up in your body. Massage helps to relax muscles so the circulation flows properly."

Improved circulation helps reduce swelling from injury and enhances the functioning of the lymphatic system, which controls immune response. "African Americans tend to have very tight bodies," Walker adds. "It comes from a combination of things like the tension and the stress we carry, and even genetics. Massage can take someone to a completely different state of mind. It's a place where you are more fluid and creative and better prepared to welcome perfect health."

Massage can also flush out wastes—such as lactic acid (which increases in the body after a rigorous workout)—from tired muscles, relieving aches and pains.

"Massage basically benefits every system of the body," Shanks says. "It increases range of motion, increases the healthiness of the muscular system, decreases blood pressure, helps to develop a stronger heart, nervous system, respiratory system, and digestive system."

Cautions

Because massage affects blood circulation, you should not get a massage if you have a fever, diarrhea, nausea, or internal bleeding. "Circulation increases and so massage can spread these conditions," Shanks explains. People with acute phlebitis, thrombosis, or varicose veins should also avoid massage because such conditions can result in blood clotting and massage can transport the blood clot to the heart or brain, increasing the risk of a stroke or heart failure. "Because of the risk of blood clots, older people should check with their doctor before getting a massage," Walker adds. People with the following conditions may receive massage, but certain body parts should be avoided during the session: in the case of high blood pressure or heart problems, no massage to the abdomen and in the case of chronic varicose veins, fractures or bruises, no massage directly over the site. Pregnant women should also check with their doctor before getting a massage. Some therapists specialize in pregnancy massage and are available through a doctor's referral.

Choosing a Therapist

Choose a massage therapist with some care. Given the vulnerability involved with being unclothed and touched by a stranger, finding a therapist you feel comfortable with is vital. "It's a blessing when a person comes to me, and I am the first person to give them a massage," Spillman says. "The first time is so crucial, so I try to give the person the best experience possible, not only so they will come back to me, but so they will see over time how beneficial massage is to their lives."

Your therapist should be attuned to your needs. If a therapist does not set aside his or her own troubles, she may massage too vigorously in a sensitive area or not rub hard enough in a place that really needs it. "A therapist must be totally aware of the client, paying attention to how the client is responding to the treatment," Spillman explains. Finding a therapist who is at peace with herself helps guarantee a peaceful experience for the client.

There are a few commonsense ways to judge whether or not a therapist is right for you. "Listen to their voice," Walker advises. "Does the person sound hectic, rushed, or on edge? That's one extreme, but the other is, does the person sound too airy and light? Look for someone who seems centered and calm and someone you feel comfortable with."

Training is also a factor in choosing a therapist. On average, massage therapists must undergo 300 to 1,000 hours of formal training to join one of the two major membership organizations, the American Massage Therapy Association (AMTA) or the Association of Bodywork and Massage Professionals (ABMP). AMTA requires members to be graduates of one of approximately sixty schools with approved curriculum or pass a national equivalency certification examination given by the national Certification Board for Therapeutic Massage and Bodywork. AMTA schools must provide a minimum 500-hour program including courses in anatomy, physiology, pathology, and hands-on massage training, plus courses in first aid, cardiopulmonary resuscitation (CPR), and professional business practices. Professional level of membership requires 500 hours of education or state massage license or certification.

But there's more to giving a good massage than training. "It's beyond education," Walker says. "What impresses me more is how long someone has been doing what they do and how they feel about what they do. Referrals from friends and family members are also a good way to gauge a therapist's experience or how well he or she aims to please."

A good therapist should be able to answer virtually any question you may have or point you toward resources for more information. "During an initial discussion or while filling out the intake form, use this time to ask any questions you may have, such as questions about the safety of massage and the various types used by the therapist," Shanks says. " 'What's your approach?' is always a good question to ask, so you will at least learn a little bit about what's going to occur in the next hour," Spillman adds.

Besides the questions and concerns you may have on that day, it is a good idea to find out ahead of time answers to questions such as: "Can I keep my underwear on?", "What kind of music do you play?", or "Do you use candles or incense to set a relaxing mood?" If you have preferences, be sure to mention them to the therapist when you set the appointment.

Cost

A typical massage session lasts thirty to sixty minutes, but might be briefer for kids, the elderly, and the ill or otherwise injured. A session can run anywhere from $30 to $100, but on average should run about $60 for an hour. Your insurer may pay for a massage session, so be sure to check before making an appointment. You can also contact a professional organization (listed below) or a local massage school for recommendations.

Can I Do it Myself?

"You can rub your own feet or hands or wherever you feel stress and discomfort and experience some relaxation," Spillman says.

"But there's nothing like the touch of another human being who, in a nurturing way, searches out your pain and brings you relief."

For Information and Referrals
American Massage Therapy Association
820 Davis St., Suite 100
Evanston, IL 60201–4444
Tel: 708–864–0123
Fax: 708–864–1178

Association of Bodywork and Massage Professionals
28677 Buffalo Park
Evergreen, CO 80439–7347
Tel: 303–674–8478
Fax: 303–674–0859

National Association of Massage Therapy
P.O. Box 1400
Westminster, CO 80030–1400
Tel: 1–800–776–6268

The Ultimate Stress Reliever—Massage

After a long day of stress, pressures, worries, and other concerns of modern life, your body and mind are crying out for relief. A great way to get that relief is through massage. Achieved with the help of a partner, this form of relaxation has been providing stress relief for centuries in many ancient cultures. Many people have found it to be a saving grace today. Here's how you can reap the benefits of massage:

First, find a quiet, clean, relaxing place. A bedroom will do; however, it is advised to administer massage on a futon-like mattress rather than a traditional mattress so the back muscles experience greater support.

When giving or receiving massage you can try one or more of the following techniques:

Effleurage: a long, gliding stroke administered with the whole hand or thumb.

Petrissage: kneading and compression motions.

Friction: consists of deep circular movements made with the thumb pads or fingertips.

Vibration: involves a very fine, rapid shaking movement.

Tapotement: consists of a series of quickly allied movements using the hand alternatively to strike or tap the muscles.

Reflexology

When Los Angeles, California-based reflexologist Martinette Jenkins goes roller skating, people think she's a wonder. It's not her skating prowess that wows them. It's her ability to heal. "I meet a lot of people roller skating, and it never fails that someone has an unbearable headache or various aches and pains that they want to get rid of." By touching the right places on their hands or feet, Jenkins magically makes the pain go away. "I can generally get rid of a headache in three to five minutes, perhaps a little longer for a migraine," says Jenkins. "They call me a miracle worker."

When Washington, D.C.-based reflexologist Njideka Olatunde first started her practice twelve years ago, she worked with senior citizens. One day, a client said she had just seen her doctor. "He told her to keep doing whatever she was doing; her cancer had been sent into remission." Cases like that make Olatunde a believer in the healing powers of reflexology. "This was actual proof to me that my work was valuable in helping people prevent illness or at least assist in their healing."

Chicago, Illinois-based reflexologist Larry Clemmons tells of a woman who came to him after visiting a podiatrist who had shaved a callus too closely. Her infected foot had turned black with gangrene. "Her medical doctor wanted to amputate the lower part of her leg," Clemmons explains. "But working in tandem with her doctor, I improved her circulation so dramatically that in the end, she lost only a toe."

Whether to heal sickness or to prevent it, reflexology is one holistic therapy that deserves more attention. The practice has roots in ancient Egypt, China, and Greece. An ancient Egyptian wall painting more than 4,000 years old shows two practitioners working the feet of two patients. Despite the extensive history of the healing art and the results that contemporary reflexologists can bring, many African Americans remain skeptical about the therapy. "African Americans are conditioned to operate from an emergency mentality rather than a preventive frame of mind," Olatunde believes. "Emergencies are covered by insurance, while preventive care is usually an out-of-pocket expense." She believes that when Health Maintenance Organizations (HMOs) start emphasizing preventive care, African Americans will be more willing to try something new.

"It's not that we can't afford to see a reflexologist," Clemmons says. "After all, we spend money to maintain our beauty." He admits, however, that an increase in health consciousness has introduced more African Americans to preventive therapies. "Most of my clients over the years have been White, but now my African American clientele is steadily increasing."

What is Reflexology?

Reflexology operates from the premise that there are 7,800 nerve endings in the feet, hands, and ears that correspond with various glands, organs, and parts of the body. "By manipulating these nerve endings, reflexologists can release tension, improve circulation and normalize body functions," says Clemmons.

All body parts, organs, and glands are associated with specific areas of the feet, hands and ears known as reflex zones. While the hands and ears contain reflexes that can be used to affect various organs, the feet are more sensitive because they are protected from the elements by shoes and socks. Therefore, the feet are the primary emphasis of the reflexologist.

In reflexology, illness and disease are caused by congestion and imbalance. By manipulating the reflex zones in the feet that correspond to various organs, reflexologists relieve congestion and imbalance. "The basic goal is to improve circulation," Olatunde explains. "When the circulation is blocked, you may experience numbness and pain. Reflexology relieves such symptoms by increasing circulation in the blocked area." Improving circulation helps move disease-causing toxins out of the affected person's system.

Modern reflexology was developed in the early twentieth century by two Americans, Dr. William Fitzgerald and Eunice Ingham. Dr. Fitzgerald developed the idea that the body is divided into ten equal zones that extend the entire length of the body from head to toe. These zones are all represented on the feet, so that stimulation of an area of the foot in one zone affects the organs, glands, or body parts that correspond to that zone. Eunice Ingham continued Dr. Fitzgerald's work by developing a detailed map of the foot, identifying each area of the foot with a corresponding organ, gland, or body part. Ingham, a physical therapist, published her extensive research in her 1938 book *Stories the Feet Can Tell.* She then founded the International Institute of Reflexology, which remains the largest training organization for reflexology, having taught over 70,000 students worldwide.

How Does it Work?

While some may consider reflexology foot massage, reflexologists are quick to differ. "Reflexology does not massage," Olatunde says. "In massage you are working with certain muscles and soft tissues, but with reflexology you are working to stimulate nerve endings. You are working with the nervous system and not the muscles."

Before a session begins, the client fills out an intake form. "This is important because it tells me their previous medical history and what they may be looking to get out of the session," Jenkins says. This is also the time when clients can ask the reflexologist any questions or concerns they may have before beginning the session. "A good reflexologist will make this time available for the client," Naillah Beraki adds.

Because reflexologists work primarily on the feet, only the feet have to be exposed. Most reflexologists ask clients to be sure that both feet are thoroughly cleaned prior to a session. "To make the client as comfortable as possible, I use a massage table and prop the feet up on pillows," Beraki says. "I also use soft music and visualizations to help a client relax." The environment should be healing, quiet, serene and inviting, Olatunde adds. "There should be no offensive odors—everything should be in a neutral state with the client in a comfortable chair or on a massage table." Before work begins, the reflexologist examines a client's feet to make sure there are no calluses, wounds, or scars that might be painful to the touch. It is important for clients to share such information during the intake section of the treatment.

Reflexologists apply pressure to reflex points in a variety of ways—rubbing, rotating, and caterpillar-like movement. Most begin by gently stroking the entire foot. The strokes are firm, so that there is no tickle even with the most sensitive of feet. Even if a client does not articulate where in the body they are experiencing discomfort, a reflexologist often knows. "Reflexologists feel for 'crystals,' a gritty feeling in nerve endings that indicates poor circulation in a particular area of the body," Olatunde explains.

A therapist knows where the client needs the most work by how the client responds to touch. For instance, when the therapist touches the big toe, a sharp pain or other irritation tells the therapist her client may be experiencing a headache because the big toe represents the temple. To relieve the headache, the reflexologist applies pressure to the big toe with the fingers and slowly works the pain away. "Reflexology works by stimulating endorphins— your body's natural pain killers—to help heal discomfort," Clemmons explains. "Therapists create alternating pressure along the reflexes of the feet, creating an endorphin response that takes away the pain." This allows the body to relax and begin to heal congestion and imbalance.

Clients may experience a variety of sensations as the reflexologist works on various parts of the foot. Any discomfort is usually brief and is felt only in areas where congestion may be blocking circulation and causing a problem. While most people report a feeling of relaxation immediately after a session, some may experience a cleansing reaction that could include a runny nose, headaches, or a mild rash. A cleansing reaction indicates that your body is trying to get rid of released congestion. Many reflexologists recommend drinking generous amounts of water to help assist this cleansing.

Best Uses

Reflexology is useful for such stress-related physical health challenges such as hypertension, lower back pain, digestive problems, fatigue, and aches and pains. "Reflexology is also wonderful for pregnant women," Beraki adds. "It helps to eliminate the swelling in the legs and feet that some pregnant women experience." But, "We are not doctors, and we do not diagnose," she says. "So practitioners should not make promises." Although many practitioners report remarkable stories of clients making dramatic recoveries, little scientific research has been conducted to ascertain the effectiveness of reflexology. "One thing is for sure," Olatunde says, "reflexology can work hand in hand with conventional medicine and enhance healing and prevention."

Cautions

There are very few cautions with reflexology, but the technique may not be advisable for some conditions. "Reflexology may cause problems for a person on a lot of toxic medication," Jenkins says. "Because reflexology releases toxins already in the system, combine those toxins with those created by some medications, and too much may be released, overrunning a person's system."

Beraki warns that people with acute swelling or redness on the bottom of the feet should avoid reflexology on the feet until their condition improves. "For such persons, working on the hands, although they are not as sensitive as the feet, can be just as effective," Clemmons says. Finally, reflexology should be used with caution in cases of pneumonia. "In the healing response more fluid is secreted into the lymph system," Clemmons says. "A person with pneumonia may not be able to expel toxins fast enough. You can work on a person with pneumonia, but it has to be brief and in tandem with a medical doctor."

While adverse reactions to reflexology are possible, they appear to be rare. "Most people benefit tremendously," Olatunde says. "Positive results can often be seen after the first session."

Choosing a Therapist

Many massage therapists, doctors, and chiropractors incorporate reflexology into their practice. "Anyone considering reflexology should know the training of their therapist," Olatunde explains. "A good reflexologist needs a minimum of 200 hours of certified training." There is currently no national license for reflexologists, although the American Reflexology Certification board has introduced a voluntary national certification program that it administers. The International Institute of Reflexology offers the oldest certification program. Until a national licensure is adopted, each state has its own rules regarding reflexologists and requirements for practicing. Contact the national associations for reflexology (see p. 175) for additional training information.

Before the session begins, ask if the reflexologist has treated other clients with your particular condition. One of the most important questions to ask is what to expect. "Make sure the therapist thoroughly explains what can be expected, and don't be shy about asking whether or not there will be any pain," Beraki says. Speaking of pain, she adds with a laugh, "I'd stay away from therapists with long fingernails."

Cost

A typical session lasts 45 to 90 minutes, and although the price ranges from $25 to $65 nationwide, it can go as high as $200. "I usually operate on a sliding scale," Jenkins says. "I don't want anyone who needs it not to be able to have a session because of money." Referrals from the International Institute of Reflexology or friends and family members are the best ways to determine if you are getting your money's worth.

Can I Do it Myself?

Virtually anyone can practice reflexology on themselves. "Older people with arthritis may have a difficult time reaching their feet, but they can work their hands, which can be just as effective," Clemmons says. "Just search out the tender spots and reflex them out with a little pressure," Jenkins adds.

Olatunde believes that at least one member of every family should know reflexology and use it as a first-aid tool. "People should take advantage of introductory reflexology classes whenever they are offered."

For Further Information and Referrals
International Institute of Reflexology
P.O. Box 12642
St. Petersburg, FL 33733–2642
Tel: 813–343–4811
Fax: 813–381–2807

American Reflexology Certification Board
P.O. Box 620607
Littleton, CO 80162
Tel: 303–933–6921

Reflexology Basics

Reflexology is a science based on the premise that the organs, limbs, and body systems, i.e., digestive, reproductive, and respiratory, are represented by the reflexes in the feet and hands. These reflexes, it is believed, are linked to pathways that, when blocked, cause imbalance and disruption in many facets of your health. Disruptions manifest themselves in emotional problems, stress, and dietary habits. When there is imbalance or blockage in the body, immune efficiencies are broken down and the body is unable to heal itself, resulting in illness. Many reflexologists believe that stress is a factor in more than 75 percent of all illness. Stress in any form prevents your own natural healing powers from working. Reflexology clears your body's natural healing powers by clearing blocked pathways. Once blocked pathways are cleared, detoxification can occur, allowing the immune system, in conjunction with other bodily functions, to reach a state of balance and heightened efficiency.

In addition to releasing tension and relaxing a patient,

reflexology has been known to help alleviate asthma and other respiratory conditions, menstrual and menopausal symptoms, sports injuries, nervous system, skin, and digestive disorders, emotional problems, back troubles, headaches and migraine headaches, and insomnia.

Vitamin and Nutrition Therapy

Barbara Dixon's father died of a heart attack at age forty-five. By the time her mother was forty-five, she had suffered four strokes. But Dixon herself has surpassed age forty-five and she's the picture of health. How has a woman whose family has fallen to so many tragedies managed to avoid the same fate?

Good nutrition. "I have to conclude that it's because I eat a variety of healthy foods and exercise," says Dixon, a registered dietitian and nutritionist who operates the Dixon Medical and Nutritional Clinic in Baton Rouge, Louisiana.

Nutritionist Lauren Swann, M.S., R.D., feels the same way. Diabetes is a major concern for Swann because it runs in her family. "Because I know I may be prone to diabetes, I can take steps like eating a properly balanced diet, avoiding processed sugars, and I can exercise, so that if diabetes hits most people in my family before they're forty, maybe it won't hit me until I'm sixty or seventy, if at all."

From the time of slavery to today, most African American nutritionists agree, our diet has gone steadily downhill. "Historically, Africans ate abundant grains, vegetables, and fruit," says Swann, president of her Philadelphia, Pennsylvania-based consulting firm, Concept Nutrition. "While Africans were not necessarily vegetarians, the meat they did eat was freshly killed and not mass-produced."

Even in slavery, the African American diet was still reasonably healthful. Along with steady rations of corn meal and occasional meat, slaves ate the fresh vegetables that they were typically allowed to grow near their quarters. Once slavery ended, though, many African Americans rushed out to enjoy foods they had long been denied. "It was as if we were saying, 'I can now have this,' when it came to eating meat," Swann says.

These early experiences still affect the way we eat. As a consultant for Headstart and WIC (Women, Infants and Children) programs, Swann has worked with families who dine at fast food restaurants three or four times a week. "Lots of our neighborhoods have fast food outlets on every corner and the produce in the grocery stores is horrible." Swann sees an overreliance on processed foods and less access to fresh fruits and vegetables as major problems for African Americans today, problems that lead to significant health challenges.

But there is hope. Improving vitamin and nutrient intake by eating a properly balanced diet is just what the doctor orders when battling an illness or trying to prevent one. "Food can be your best medicine or your worst enemy," says Brooklyn, New York-based Kamau Kukayi, M.D., who specializes in naturopathic and Chinese herbal remedies.

"We don't have any proof that if you eat ten cups of broccoli a day, you won't get cancer," Swann says. "Science doesn't work that way. But all the odds seem to suggest that eating certain foods either prevents many diseases from ever developing, minimizes the risks of getting a disease, or at least defers when a disease may start."

What is Vitamin and Nutrition Therapy?
With the growth of nutritional science in the twentieth century, it's no longer a question that certain foods increase your risk for certain diseases. Too much fat (saturated animal fat in particular) heightens your risk for heart disease and breast and colon cancers. Too much refined flour and sugar and too little fiber can cause

digestive and bowel disorders like constipation and hemorrhoids. Too much salt can raise blood pressure. On one hand, vitamin and nutrition therapy involves correcting these excesses so that people consume a diet that is in proper balance.

But there's more. "We also know that some medical conditions are caused by vitamin deficiencies," says Cleveland, Ohio-based Ronald Casselberry, M.D. "Vitamin and nutrition therapy means finding out which nutrients a person may be deficient in and then working to give the body what it needs." At The Progressive Pain Relief and Medical Health Center, owned and operated by Dr. Casselberry and his brother, massage therapist Michael Casselberry, treatment is a mix of both conventional and nutritional therapies. "Before I use medicine, I first try to find out if there are any nutrient deficiencies or any absence of vitamins, minerals, or enzymes. For example, sometimes a person who has arthritis lacks essential fatty acids." For such patients, Casselberry may recommend natural flaxseed oil, which helps to lubricate the joints, instead of costly anti-inflammatory medication, which may have unwanted side effects.

Practitioners use vitamin and nutrition therapy to cure illness as well as to prevent it. Dr. Kukayi believes a balanced diet plus supplements like multivitamins or specific supplements for individual patients can help ward off a number of diseases. "It's a fact that foods rich in antioxidants and other vitamins and minerals help to fight free radicals before they can cause disease," Dr. Kukayi says.

"Your body will take care of you if you take care of it," says Pearleen Jackson, N.D., who is based in Philadelphia, Pennsylvania.

How Does it Work?

Vitamin and nutrition therapy is a broad-based approach to prevention and healing. For example, some practitioners use nutrients, trace minerals, enzymes, vitamin supplements, organic foods, and juicing to treat cancer and AIDS. The enzymes help break down cancer cells and improve digestion; proper nutrients offer the body nutritional support. "But no one puts cancer into remission just by eating right and taking herbs," Dr. Jackson says. "You have to believe in what you are doing and keep yourself free of anxiety, impatience, and frustration."

Dr. Casselberry agrees. "A person has to be highly motivated to undergo such a program because you have to break bad habits, shop for healthful foods, and read food labels."

One way Dr. Jackson determines the deficiencies in a client's diet is a live-cell analysis. "The client comes in; I prick their finger and examine a drop of blood under the microscope to determine the nutrient status of the cells, immune function, and the presence or absence of yeast, parasites, and bacteria," Dr. Jackson says. "I can also see if the kidneys are functioning properly by the presence or absence of crystals in the blood. From this overall analysis, I can see what a person needs and can recommend a nutritional program tailored to meet those needs."

But one of the best ways to understand what a person needs, according to Dr. Jackson, is to listen to what they say. "The person's family history—whether fibroids or drugs and alcohol run in the family—is important since we are what we come from. Most of us follow parental diets; we eat foods based upon the foods our parents reared us on. For instance, my mother ate pig's feet because her mother had fixed it for her. But there is a high incidence of stroke in the family, so she decided to change her diet to avoid the fat and reduce her risk of similar diseases. She lived to be eighty-six years old, outliving many family members."

"If you are deficient in certain nutrients, it will appear as certain symptoms," Dr. Casselberry says. Skin and vision problems may indicate a vitamin A deficiency; blisters in the mouth and scurvy may indicate a vitamin C deficiency; and anemia could indicate a lack of iron. To address such problems, Dr. Casselberry typically reviews the client's diet. "Having the client fill out a nutritional sheet that outlines their average daily diet helps us define what the source of the problem could be," he says. "Then recommendations can be made to correct any shortcomings."

Best Uses

Vitamin and nutrition therapy can be useful for a variety of diseases and conditions, both acute and chronic. "I've seen patients suffering from diabetes and hypertension who were eating high-fat diets with no variety and few vegetables, fruits, or whole grains reverse illness and drop their dependence on medications, thanks to a dietary change," Dr. Kukayi says.

Jifunza Wright-Carter, M.D., a Chicago, Illinois-based family physician who specializes in holistic medicine, has had similar experiences. "I've had patients with malignant (life-threatening) hypertension reverse it with food and lifestyle changes," she says. "We emphasize eating foods that are low in fat and high in fiber and foods that are fresh, not processed."

The therapy is useful as a preventive measure. For example, the common cold is an excellent candidate for nutritional and vitamin therapy. Practitioners recommend taking 3,000 milligrams to 4,000 milligrams a day of vitamin C and supplementing that with the herb echinacea at the first stages of a cold. The vitamin C dosage should not be taken at once—it can cause diarrhea that way—but spread out throughout the day. Because vitamin C is water-soluble and not absorbed into fatty tissue, any excess will leave the body in the urine. Nervousness and irritability could indicate that the person needs more vitamin B. "The easiest way to put them back in balance is to give them vitamin-rich kale, turnip, and mustard greens," Dr. Jackson says. "Certain foods—like radishes, green peas, lemons, and apple cider vinegar—break up mucus in the lungs and large intestines, helping you to breathe better and relieving pneumonia," she adds. "Fatty foods, cold foods, and cold drinks cause constriction and weaken the lungs and large intestine. Garlic, brown rice, and melons strengthen the lungs and large intestine."

While all the vitamins and minerals a person needs are available in a well-balanced diet—in other words, fresh fruits and vegetables; whole grains like millet, quinoa, and whole wheat; meat, sugar and dairy only in sparing amounts—vitamin supplementation is an acceptable way of getting nutrients you may feel you are missing.

Cautions

Unlike water-soluble vitamins, which pass right through you and leave the body in the urine, fat-soluble vitamins (A, D, E, and K) accumulate in your body, especially if you are overweight. High doses of these vitamins can be toxic. For example, doses of vitamin A above 20,000 international units (IU) can cause severe pressure in the head. Be careful to adhere to label recommendations or the advice of an experienced and properly trained professional.

Treating serious illnesses like cancer, diabetes, or AIDS with nutritional and vitamin supplements may require megadosing, which could in some cases mean taking 100 pills a day. Such high doses should always be taken under the guidance of a nutritional therapist or physician.

Avoid vitamins made from ingredients that the body may not use as readily as vitamins extracted from food sources. "Look for supplements that are food-grade vitamins, which means they were taken from a plant, and while processing, the nutrients were not heated over room temperature," Dr. Casselberry advises. "Above 110 degrees, enzymes and vitamins break down and lose their nutritional value." That's also why it's important to store them in a cool, dry place. "Food is most nutritious when it is raw," elaborates vegetarian and herbalist Yemi Bates-Jones, wellness counselor at the Cottonwood Health Spa in Cottonwood, Alabama. Bates-Jones recommends eating foods closer to their natural state. That means fresh fruits and vegetables; steaming instead of endless boiling; whole grains rather than refined wheat and rice. Move away from salt and season instead with onion, garlic, lemon juice, and nature's many herbs and spices.

Avoid fruits and vegetables that are not in season. When your grocer carries fruits and vegetables in low quantities, chances are these foods were grown outside the United States, where weaker pesticide laws can mean that produce imported to America can carry high levels of pesticide residues. In the fall and winter, as the plants lose their leaves and their energy goes underground, eat root vegetables like carrots, rhubarbs, turnips, and radishes, Dr. Jackson advises. As energy moves up in the spring and summer, eat squash, cabbage, turnip greens, and mustard greens. "Eat more live foods (uncooked foods, such as fruits, salads, and greens) during the warmer months. You need more heat in the winter and less in the spring and summer."

Shopping for organic produce at health food stores or local farmers' markets ensures a crop with integrity, because organic foods must meet strict controls. Organic foods come with the guarantee that no toxic pesticides were used on the plants or in the soil. If you buy your produce from the grocery store, Dr. Jackson suggests, soak fruits and vegetables for ten minutes in a sink full of cold water and vinegar (a capful is enough). This helps to rinse off any toxic residues.

Choosing a Therapist

Word of mouth is the number one way to locate a nutritionist or holistic health practitioner who can evaluate your diet and help you improve eating habits and choose supplements. The American Dietetic Association (see p. 184) can also help you find a practitioner in your area.

When you meet a therapist, observe him or her carefully to see if they practice what they preach. Is his skin healthy? Are his eyes clear? How is her posture? "A lot of people give lip service to good health, but make sure your therapist is actually practicing it," Dr. Jackson advises. "You can't help anyone else until you've helped yourself."

Ask where your therapist received his or her training. Inquire about licenses and degrees in nutrition or another holistic therapy. Ask the practitioner about his or her philosophy on healing. "If you want a holistic healer, then don't choose a physician who is not open to holistic alternatives," Dr. Casselberry adds.

If you are experiencing symptoms that may indicate a vitamin deficiency, ask exactly what you can do to resolve the problem. After examining your dietary habits, a therapist should be able to make specific recommendations. Make sure you understand their suggestions and know exactly how certain changes will help your condition.

Cost

Depending on whether you require any blood-work analysis or simply a review of nutritional habits, the average cost of seeking nutritional advice ranges from $50 to $100. Vitamins and supplements are relatively inexpensive, ranging from $5 to $20, depending on the supplement and the number of pills (usually thirty, sixty, or ninety per bottle). With serious illnesses such as cancer, diabetes, or AIDS, supplements can be expensive if you require frequent refills. Still, vitamin supplements and dietary changes typically prove to be less expensive and safer alternatives to pharmaceuticals in the long run.

Organic produce in a health food grocery store can cost 10 to 50 percent more than produce in traditional grocery stores, but they are guaranteed free of pesticides and are usually grown with soil-enhancing fertilizers. Look for farm-raised chicken and fish at some health food stores if you include those items in your diet.

Many health food stores are not traditionally located in urban African American communities. You may have to go a little further to a suburban community, but getting organic, healthful food is worth the trip. If transportation is a problem, why not start a food co-op in your very own neighborhood? For more information, contact the Center for Cooperatives at the University of Wisconsin at Madison. The National Cooperatives Bank provides funding for co-op initiatives.

Can I Do it Myself?

Treating serious illness without guidance is never advisable. "You have to find someone who knows what they are doing," Dr. Jackson says. "Your health is not something you can afford to experiment with." However, minor illnesses like colds can be treated successfully with little professional intervention once you have learned what works for you. Consulting a holistic practitioner who can point you in the right direction is always beneficial.

After working with a nutritionist and evaluating your eating habits, improving them is certainly something that only you can do. "Not only can you do it yourself, if you listen to your body, it will continuously tell you what it needs," Dr. Jackson adds.

For More Information

American Dietetic Association
216 West Jackson Blvd., Suite 800
Chicago, IL 60606–6995
(800) 877–1600

American Association of Nutrition Consultants
1641 East Sunset Rd.
Suite B-117
Las Vegas, NV 89119
(709) 361–1132

Center for Cooperatives
University of Wisconsin at Madison
230 Taylor Hall
427 Lorch St.

Madison, WI 53706
608–262–3981

National Cooperatives Bank
1401 Eye St., NW
Washington, D.C. 20005
202–336–7687

Cooperative Development Foundation
1401 New York Ave.
Suite 1100
Washington, D.C. 20005
202–638–6222

Making Wise Food Choices

You've probably seen the U.S. Department of Agriculture's (USDA) Food Guide Pyramid on the back of your favorite cereal box. It gives five food groups and the number of daily servings we should eat from each group: six to eleven servings of grains; three to five servings of vegetables; two to four servings of fruit; two to three servings of dairy products; and two to three servings of meat, fish, poultry, beans, nuts, and eggs.

Some critics say the USDA recommendations don't go far enough—that the Food Guide Pyramid delivers too much fat and cholesterol, an overabundance of protein, and exposure to antibiotics fed to dairy cattle. The Physicians' Committee for Responsible Medicine, an organization comprised of some of the nation's leading medical authorities, recommends a different eating plan. The plan stresses four food groups— grains, legumes (beans), vegetables, and fruits. Under this plan, meat and dairy products lose their status as essential sources of nutrients.

So how does the Physicians' Committee plan measure up? Pretty well. Grains, legumes, fruits, and vegetables contain carbohydrates, protein, fiber, and essential vitamins and minerals. Foods in these groups provide energy from complex carbohydrates and plenty of fiber that keeps you regular, helps to prevent colon cancer, and lowers low-density lipoprotein blood cholesterol levels. The combined benefits of less total fat, no animal fat, fewer contaminants, more fiber, and more cancer-fighting nutrients make restricting your diet to these four food groups attractive indeed.

Whichever dietary plan you choose, you can't go wrong by making grains, vegetables, and fruits a centerpiece of your diet:

- Try to get about half of your daily calories from grains, recommends the Physicians' Committee. Whole grains are the way to go. They're much better for you than refined grains, which lose many of their nutrients during processing. That means select 100 percent whole-wheat over white bread, brown rice over white rice, and natural pastas over the bleached-out stuff on your supermarket shelves. The grain group also includes corn, oatmeal, rye, oats, millet, barley, buckwheat, and quinoa. All of those choices deliver lots of fiber, complex carbohydrates, important vitamins, and protein.

- Fruits and vegetables, like grains, are loaded with carbohydrates, fiber, minerals, and are excellent sources of vitamins A and C, which are immune system boosters. Fruits and vegetables are also naturally low in fat (especially when you lay off the oily salad dressing!). The USDA recommends eating at least five servings of fruits and vegetables daily. Eating seven or more servings provides additional protection against cancer, according to research from the National Cancer Institute.

Essential Vitamins and Nutrients

Vitamin A—Maintains vision, bones, hair, teeth, glands, skin, the reproductive system, and helps wounds heal. RDA: 2.4 milligrams for women and 3 milligrams for men.

Vitamin D—Allows the body to absorb calcium and phosphorus, helps the nervous system function by regulating muscle and nerve function. RDA: 5 micrograms for men and women, 10 micrograms for teens, young children, and pregnant women.

Vitamin E—Ensures function of the immune and endocrine systems and sex glands. Prevents hardening of the arteries. RDA: 8 milligrams for women and 10 milligrams for men and pregnant and nursing women.

Vitamin K—Assists kidney function, bone metabolism, and blood clotting. RDA: 65 micrograms for women and 80 micrograms for men.

Vitamin B_1—Assists nervous system function. Promotes increased function of metabolism to burn fat and aids digestion. RDA: 1.1 milligrams for women, 1.5 milligrams for men.

Vitamin B_2—Helps release energy to cells; helps build red blood cells. Is useful for proper function of nerves, eyes and adrenal glands. RDA: 1.3 milligrams for women and 1.7 milligrams for men, 1.6 milligrams for pregnant women.

Vitamin B_6—Forms red blood cells, promotes nerve function, supports immune system function. Is needed for protein and carbohydrate metabolism. RDA: women, 1.6 milligrams and 2 milligrams for men, 2.2 milligrams for pregnant women.

Vitamin B_{12}—Helps make red blood cells; builds genetic

material needed by cells; converts food to energy. RDA: Adults 2 micrograms, 2.2 micrograms for pregnant women.

Vitamin C—Helps bones and teeth grow, binds cells together, helps resist infection, helps heal cuts and wounds, is needed for blood clotting. RDA: Adults 60 milligrams, 70 milligrams for pregnant women.

Folate, Folic Acid—Needed to produce DNA ribonucleic acid (RNA), and blood cells; prevents neural tube defects; helps prevent fatal coronary artery disease. RDA: 400 micrograms for men and women.

Calcium—Needed for bone and teeth growth and maintenance. Enables heart and other muscle contraction. RDA: 1,200 milligrams for adults, 800 for children.

Iron—Strengthens immune system function; is essential to making hemoglobin (the ingredient in blood that carries oxygen) and myoglobin (the blood ingredient that stores oxygen in muscles). RDA: Adults 10 milligrams, 15 milligrams for premenopausal women, and 30 milligrams for pregnant women.

Potassium—In conjunction with sodium and chloride potassium assists nerve impulse transmission, muscle contractions, regulates heartbeat; is needed for proper function of protein, carbohydrate, and insulin secretion. May provide some protection against heart disease, stroke, and hypertension. RDA: 2,000 milligrams.

Holistic Dentistry

You know about acupuncture, herbology, homeopathy, and other alternative medical practices. But did you know that some maverick dentists are putting alternatives where your mouth is?

These dental health providers—known as biological or holistic dentists—believe that what's going on in the oral cavity can affect a patient's overall health and play a major role in a person's mental, physical and spiritual well-being.

"We look at the mouth as being an indicator for what may be going on in the body," says Andrea Brockman, D.D.S., a former nurse who runs a holistic dental practice with her husband in Philadelphia, Pennsylvainia. "When we see patients in our dental office, we're not just interested in fixing their teeth. We look at their entire body because there are diseases that can have an effect on the mouth and afflictions in the mouth that can have an effect on the rest of the body."

For people who live a holistic lifestyle, this approach to dentistry fits the bill. Dyane Boyd, thirty-eight, of Philadelphia, Pennsylvania, decided to visit a biological dentist when she started having earaches and unusual pains in her mouth.

"[My family uses] body workers. We use some homeopathic medicine. We use macrobiotic counseling. When I noticed the pain in my mouth, I decided to finally choose a holistic practitioner to treat my teeth," she says.

Boyd's initial examination was more involved than appointments with her former dentist.

"My new dentist asked me to fill out this rather lengthy questionnaire that took me about an hour to complete. Then she asked me questions about my health and lifestyle," Boyd says. Her new dentist even looked at her posture to check for TMJ (temporomandibular joint syndrome), the malalignment of the teeth, muscles, and jaws.

According to Stephen Odell, D.D.S., a member of the American Academy of Biological Dentistry, this kind of examination is typical among biological dentists.

"I look at areas in the face to see if there are wrinkles or signs there to help me determine the health of the patient's organs," says Dr. Odell, who is based in Carmel Valley, California. "I look at their eyes . . . I also read their tongue. Tongue reading is very important because it reveals the health of the person's system."

Odell goes a step further by incorporating his knowledge of other alternative therapies, such as Chinese medicine and iridology, to ascertain and treat other potential health problems.

Biological dentists tend to recommend natural remedies for treating most dental conditions. "In alternative dentistry you'd recommend a baking soda-peroxide mixture as a brushing medium for cleaning teeth rather than a sweet-tasting gel," says Dr. Odell. "A toothpaste with a baking soda base will lower the mouth's acidity and kill off the unwanted organisms at the gum level." Biological dentists avoid recommending toothpaste with fluoride or fluoride treatments because they believe that it's toxic to the system.

If the patient has a toothache, the biological dentist is more apt to give the patient echinacea and goldenseal than to prescribe antibiotics. Gum disease and many other oral health problems may be treated by altering the patient's diet. Similar to their traditional cohorts, however, biological dentists do pull teeth. The difference is that they may use a local anesthetic that's nonallergic or one that contains no preservatives.

One of the primary differences—and the issue that causes the most tension—between conventional and biological dentistry is the holistic practitioner's position on mercury amalgams or silver fillings, which they believe are toxic to the system.

According to *Alternative Medicine: The Definitive Guide* by the Burton Goldberg Group (Future Medicine Publishing, 1994), one of the dangers of amalgam fillings—fillings that are 50 percent mercury mixed with other metals—is that they release corroded metals into the system that can then be absorbed into the root of the tooth, mouth, and bone as well as into the connective tissues of the jaw and nervous system.

Dr. Brockman says that studies indicate that the fillings also release elemental mercury vapor each time a patient drinks or chews hot or acidic foods. Those vapors are inhaled or swallowed, which can lead to mercury toxicity with symptoms such as insomnia, chronic headaches, adrenal disease, and cancer.

Hazel J. Harper, D.D.S., president of the National Dental Association and assistant professor at Howard University's Dental School, says that the concerns regarding mercury fillings are unfounded.

"There has been no real hard conclusive scientific data that would cause any member of the dental profession to feel that he or she has the right to say that fillings, which contain several alloys including mercury, are toxic or harmful," says Dr. Harper. She says her assertion is supported by studies done by The Cancer Institute, The World Health Organization, the National Institutes of Health, and other national organizations.

The very fact that mercury has a negative effect on the environment, however, is reason enough for some dentists to avoid using the material in their practice altogether. Instead, most biological dentists use porcelain or a composite resin—materials that are less toxic—to fill a tooth.

"The problem with mercury is that it affects people in different ways, so you really can't scientifically prove that it causes disease," says Lovell Farris, D.D.S., who is one of fewer than a handful of African American dentists practicing this form of dentistry.

"But it's also correct to say that there's no proof that says it does *not* cause disease either," says the Detroit, Michigan-based dentist. "From a circumstantial point of view, there's ample evidence which points to the fact that mercury seems to be toxic in every other environment except the mouth."

So why wouldn't it be toxic in your mouth as well? Walter Beckley, thirty-nine, of Richton Park, Illinois, decided not to take any chances.

"I had been told by someone that there was a big problem with having mercury fillings in my mouth and that the mercury could cause toxicity throughout the body. So I started investigating," Beckley says. "Most of the traditional dentists I talked to told me that the mercury in my mouth wasn't a problem . . . But knowing that mercury is a highly toxic material, I decided that what the traditional dentists were telling me . . . just didn't make any sense." That was ten years ago. Beckley has been going to holistic dentists every since.

How can you find a biological dentist in your town? Check out advertisements in your local newspaper or comb the pages of your community's alternative magazines. Seldom will you find the word "biological" or "holistic" behind a dentist's name. Look for advertisements that boast a "mercury-free" practice.

Farris says whether or not you decide to switch from your conventional dentist to a holistic one, you are ultimately responsible for your dental health. "I think that what people need to do is get informed about health issues in general and learn how the whole body is connected," he says. "Find out who's practicing alternative medicine in your community. Read magazines devoted to alternative methods." And find a good health provider, he says, "a chiropractor or physician who understands the connection between this field and the overall health field—someone who knows that an unhealthy mouth represents an unhealthy body." Then put your money where your mouth is.

For a list of biological or holistic dentists in your town, call the following resources:

American Academy of Biological Dentistry
408-659-5385

Holistic Dental Association
303-259-1091

International Academy of Oral Medicine and Toxicology
407-298-2450

 ## Meditation's Healing Energy (by Kellye Davis)

For the first seventeen years of my life, I (probably like most people) identified strongly with my reflection in the mirror and ultimately with my physical body, particularly my face. But during my teenage years, life presented me with a very powerful lesson about my true identity.

The lesson came from an unlikely source—the family dog. I didn't know that our dog was sick with a brain tumor, and when I went to hug him as I normally did, the pain in his head was so great, he snapped. The bite left a scar on my left cheek. Little did I know that this unfortunate incident would fuel my spiritual journey far into my adulthood.

Prior to the accident, I was an outgoing teenager, caught up in the dramas of teenage life. On the threshold of womanhood, I toyed with the fantasies that most teenagers embrace, like going to the prom, getting on the cheerleading squad, and landing a date with Mr. Fine. In fact, my interest in the opposite sex was quite pronounced. I took great care in looking good in order to be noticed. My looks meant a lot to me.

After the accident, all of that changed. An inner shift took place. It was like a wall emerged between me and the outside world. A part of me wanted to hide—to hide my face, to hide my existence.

Still, although I was self-conscious about my scar, life went on—and so did the lessons I was to learn. Somewhere in my heart I knew I had to find a new clarity, a new reality, a new vision where my worldly eyes had no bearing and the physical world no dominion. My soul egged me on.

After graduating from college, I met a woman who was a spiritualist and heavily into the holistic and spiritual arts. One day while I was visiting her, she had a vision and told me that all of my answers and healing awaited me in meditation, and that she would take me to a place where I could learn how to meditate. And she did.

So there I was. My initial experience with meditation wasn't so easy. Actually, the whole process seemed quite difficult in the beginning, and I resisted. The practice of getting still by holding your posture in an upright position, breathing deeply with your mantra, and paying no attention to distracting thoughts and sometimes overwhelming emotions was difficult to do all at the same time. But, as I began to study meditation and experience it more and more, I learned that meditation was truly an act that bridged the physical world and the spiritual world. The practice of getting still through prescribed techniques and going beyond the chatter of my mind ultimately led me to a peaceful, thoughtless state.

I could see and feel an inner awareness developing. An inner eye within me began to show me things about myself. I would see images of my face and the scar, and it would dissolve right in front of me. I began to see shifts in myself, and how I saw myself in the physical world. Through meditation, I started to see that I was not the physical body I so desperately identified myself with. I was so much more.

As I went deeper and deeper into meditation, I began seeing numerous lights within me. Some were bright, some were dull, some were steady, while others twinkled. I began contemplating the scientific fact that when you break down physical matter to its most minute form, it becomes energy, it becomes light! Voilà! So there it was.

I began reading spiritual texts by my meditation teacher and other great meditation teachers, and they all expounded on the fact that the human body is just a shell for the divine light, the soul. Our true home is beyond the body. This was becoming real for me.

As I continued to meditate, I began to notice something magical happening to my physical body. My scar began melting away, rearranging itself, reinventing itself, as I drew closer to this new awareness. Through my own experience, I began to see how the body, which is physical matter, could be healed, transformed, and transmitted to higher states of consciousness by freeing up the mind and merging into this mindless state—the field of creation, the field of light. I realized how my physical body has been and I've also come to realize that who I really am is beyond the body—and beyond the boundaries of this world.

» PART THREE «

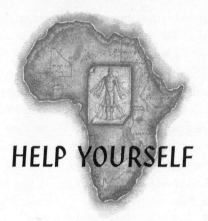

HELP YOURSELF

This section of the book describes holistic approaches to more than three dozen health problems, from allergies to yeast infections. For each health problem, we explain how you can apply some of the healing methods described in Part II of the book. The focus is on hands-on techniques and practices that you can do yourself.

Each entry:
- defines the health problem
- gives brief statistics on how prevalent the problem is among African Americans (when available)
- describes holistic approaches to treating the problem
- explains smart prevention strategies

Many of the illnesses outlined in this section are very serious, some even life-threatening. Be sure to discuss any alternative treatments, especially herbal remedies, with your physician first.

Allergies

If you're constantly sneezing around dogs and cats or get a hideous rash after eating strawberries, chances are you have an allergy. Allergies are an exaggerated response of the immune system to allergens—substances such as pollen, mold, house-dust mites, animal dander, insect bites and stings, feathers, poisonous plants, foods (especially shellfish, strawberries, nuts) or food ingredients, or drugs (such as penicillin). The immune system cannot tell if the allergens are good or bad for the body, so it releases histamines (chemicals) to attack the allergens. Histamines produce symptoms of allergies. If you have respiratory allergies, including hay fever, you will most likely experience congestion, runny nose, itchy watery eyes, itchy throat or mouth, wheezing, coughing, headache, drowsiness, and sneezing. Now if you have food allergies, you might have hives (red, itchy patches on skin), swollen lips and skin around your eyes, stomach cramps, diarrhea, nausea, vomiting, congestion, dizziness, sweating, or faintness. Skin contact with an allergen (such as household cleansers) can cause dermatitis. Most allergic reactions aren't serious, but some can be fatal, such as anaphylactic shock, commonly triggered by certain foods, insect stings and drugs (see also *Asthma*).

Statistics

Allergies are very common, affecting millions of Americans of all races. Approximately 15 percent of Americans are allergic to insect stings; 1 percent have true food allergies (not food sensitivities); and about 20 million suffer from hay fever. Hay fever is often—but not always—a childhood illness that subsides with age. Allergies tend to run in families, and people who have one allergic condition (such as hay fever) tend to have others (such as dermatitis).

Treatments

ACUPRESSURE

To get relief from symptoms including headaches, sneezing, and itching eyes, find the highest spot of the area between the thumb and index finger, and rub firmly for one minute. Repeat on your other hand. **Do not press this point if you are pregnant.** To strengthen your immune system and keep colds at bay, find the spot on top of your forearm between your two arm bones, two finger-widths from your wrist. Firmly massage this area with a deep circular motion of your thumb.

AROMATHERAPY

Add 1 drop essential oil of lavender to 1 teaspoon carrier oil or lotion. Massage into your skin over your sinuses on either side of your nose once a day. Dilute 1 drop of essential oil of inula in 1 teaspoon of jojoba or sweet almond oil. Rub into your skin over your sinuses once a day.

AYURVEDIC MEDICINE

For hay fever, apply 3 drops of warm ghee, or clarified butter, to your nostrils with the tip of your pinkie finger three times a day. To make ghee, melt 2 pounds of unsalted butter in a heavy saucepan. When it starts to boil, reduce heat to a simmer. Simmer until golden and foam disappears. Stir occasionally until curds sink to the bottom. Ghee is ready when curds turn a light tan color. Cool and strain into a container. Throw away curds.

HERBAL REMEDIES

Try horehound (in a tea bag, hard candy, or cough lozenge), aspidosperma, and cabbage to soothe your bronchial passages and help to clear mucus. Also good for sore throats are poke root and echinacea. Echinacea can be brewed as a tea (1 teaspoon in a cup of water, taken three times a day), or as a tincture (30 drops taken four times a day), or in capsules (follow label for dosage). Infuse some chamomile, elder flower, eyebright, garlic, goldenrod, nettle, and yarrow to help clear congestion.

HOMEOPATHY

With Apis Mellifica 30C (Honeybee) being the best remedy, Allium Cepa 30C (Red Onion) is great for allergy symptoms involving sneezing, runny nose, and watery eyes. If your allergy brings symptoms that cause the eyes to burn and water, use Euphracia 30C (Eyebright).

MIND-BODY

Staying active can help control allergies, which are often aggravated by stress. Jogging, brisk walking, or swimming are particularly good activities to keep you calm, cool, and collected. You can also combat stress and allergies with daily yoga and meditation. Some poses to try: cobra, boat, knee squeeze, standing sun, seated sun.

NUTRITION AND DIET

Get plenty of vitamin C combined with bioflavonoids (an organic chemical compound found in citrus fruits) to control a runny nose or alleviate congestion by eating citrus fruits or taking supplements. Vitamins A and pantothenic acid (vitamin B_5), which is found in red meat, dark turkey meat, salmon, wheat bran, brewer's yeast, brown rice, beans, nuts, corn, peas, sweet potatoes, and eggs boost the immune system. You might also try licorice or beta-carotene supplements to alleviate allergy symptoms—be sure to read labels for recommended dosage.

Prevention

If you find yourself prone to certain allergies, take these steps to avoid them. Vacuum floors and carpets daily to eliminate indoor pollutants. Wear sunglasses to reduce pollen exposure. Use air conditioning in warm weather to prevent exposure to allergens.

Use ionizers to remove pollen, dust, and other airborne allergens; get a high-efficiency air cleaner to remove pollen and mold spores. Keep pets outside when possible and bathe them frequently to reduce dander. Avoid foods and chemicals that induce an allergic reaction, such as yellow food dye No. 5 and gum arabic.

Arthritis

At one time or another, you've probably heard an older family member refer to his or her friend, Arthur. That familiar friend they're speaking of is probably arthritis. Osteoarthritis (degenerative arthritis) is the most common form of arthritis. It occurs when the smooth layers of cartilage that act as a pad between the bones in a joint become thin, frayed, or worn. Symptoms include pain, swelling, stiffness, and limited movement in affected joints. Usually hereditary, arthritis can also result from years of wear and tear.

Rheumatoid arthritis is a chronic inflammatory autoimmune disorder. Symptoms include pain, stiffness, swelling, deformity, and permanent loss of function in the affected joints. Rheumatoid arthritis may also cause fatigue, weakness, and loss of appetite.

Statistics
Nearly 4 million African Americans (more than 12 percent of Blacks) are affected by arthritis. African Americans are more likely than Whites to experience higher rates of limitations in daily activities and in employment due to arthritis.

Treatments

ACUPRESSURE
To alleviate pain in the neck, use both of your thumbs to press the points below the base of your skull, about 2 inches from the middle of your neck (GB 20) for one minute.

AROMATHERAPY
Use 6 drops each of rosemary and chamomile essential oils to add to 4 ounces of a carrier oil (almond, avocado, sesame). Massage into joints for relief from pain and stiffness.

AYURVEDIC MEDICINE
Rub warm sesame oil on sore joints one or two times a day, then take a hot shower that lasts twenty to sixty minutes. Also, try adding cayenne, ginger, or cinnamon to your diet.

CHINESE MEDICINE
Acupuncture provides relief from symptoms, especially in the hips, knees, feet, and hands. Some of the most commonly used herbs that practitioners use are: bupleuri root, licorice, and Chinese skullcap for inflammation caused by rheumatoid arthritis. For osteoarthritis, pubescebt angelica root, ledebouriellua root, timospora stem, and cinnamon twigs can be helpful if the arthritis is caught in early stages. You should consult a qualified practitioner for additional information on specific quantities.

CHIROPRACTIC
Chiropractic care is particularly effective for osteoarthritis because it eases pain through manipulation of the spine and the joints.

HERBAL THERAPY
The following are a few herbal remedies that holistic practitioners suggest: Drink powdered willow bark or meadowsweet as a tea. Use comfrey cream, wintergreen (menthol) oil, linseed oil, juniper oil, or borage oil as rubs for aching joints. Hot compresses of angelica root tincture, meadowsweet tincture, or diluted chickweed tincture help alleviate symptoms. Ginger (add 1 teaspoon ginger to 1 cup water; simmer fifteen minutes; drink three times

a day) may relieve rheumatoid arthritis; devil's claw decoction or tablets can help, too.

HOMEOPATHY

The pains and stiffness of arthritis benefit greatly from Rhus Toxicodendron 6C (Poison Ivy). It is also good for ailments from strains, overlifting, and rheumatic pains. Another good remedy is Bryonia 6C (Wild Hops), which helps when the pain is accompanied by swollen, red, tender joints.

MASSAGE

Massage helps to relax muscles so the circulation flows properly. In turn, improved circulation helps reduce swelling, which is common in arthritis. Even more beneficial, it increases range of motion. Massage some vegetable oil gently around sore joints, making small circles with your fingertips for three to five minutes a day. For rheumatoid arthritis, gently use your palms or fingertips (with oil or cream on them) to lightly stroke around sore joints toward your heart five to ten minutes a day.

MIND-BODY

Keep your body moving with daily exercise. Try spending some time in a pool or other body of water to strengthen muscles and increase circulation without stressing the body. Or put one foot in front of the other and walk your way to better health (twenty to thirty minutes a day). For a do-it-yourself massage, gently rub a light cream or oil into your skin, stroking muscles and tissues around sore areas, in the direction of the heart; or apply pressure over the area with a tennis ball. Daily imagery, biofeedback, meditation, stretch-based relaxation, or yoga can be helpful in controlling pain. For imagery, try to visualize in your mind the joint pain and what you think it looks like. Turn it into a liquid form and picture it flowing down your leg to your feet and floating far away. Do this for ten to twenty minutes twice a day.

NUTRITION AND DIET

Make sure to get plenty of omega-3 fatty acids (from fish oil) that lubricate joints and may block the body's production of prostaglandins, which trigger inflammation. Also, eat a diet rich in whole grains, fresh vegetables, and fruits. Try eliminating the nightshade family of foods (potatoes, tomatoes, eggplant, peppers, paprika, cayenne, and tobacco) for a month and see if you can detect any change in symptoms—the alkaloids in these foods are believed to inhibit repair of collagen, a protein that helps form cartilage. You'll want to supplement your diet with boron or the amino acid methionine, which create and repair cartilage. Pantothenic acid (vitamin B_5) helps prevent and alleviate arthritis. Vitamins E, C, B_6, B_1, B_{12}, A, zinc, and copper taken in multivitamin supplements also help reduce pain and swelling, and build and repair connective tissue. Also, drinking two glasses of black cherry juice twice a day can help relieve pain; or try making juice from pineapple, apple, ginger, broccoli, or spinach for rheumatoid arthritis.

Prevention

Try to maintain a normal body weight for your age, height, and body frame. You'll want to avoid fried foods, butter, red meat, cheese, and nuts. Eliminate refined sugars, margarine, preserved meat, and refined foods. Avoid Aspartame, an artificial sweetener that causes joint pain in some.

 ## Testimonial

You won't catch anyone calling Louise Rice of Philadelphia, Pennsylvania, an old lady. Rice, sixty-three, suffers from arthritis, as do both of her siblings. But Rice is pain-free and they're not, thanks to chiropractic, massage, and herbal therapy. She visits her chiropractor three times a week, eats organic fruits and vegetables and fish and chicken; "juices" every morning; takes goldenseal, vitamin C, and ginseng; and has frequent colon cleansings. "My chiropractor helps to keep me mobile. My sister had knee replacement surgery and my brother is bedridden," says Rice. "I feel like I'm forty, and expect to live to 100."

Asthma

If you've ever run in a race or walked up a steep flight of stairs, you know what it feels like to be short of breath. Imagine if that's how it felt every time you took a breath! That's what someone having an attack experiences. Asthma is a chronic respiratory disease in which constriction or spasms of the airways are caused by allergy, tobacco smoke, animal dander, pollen, air pollution, lung infection, or stress, resulting in a tightening of the chest and difficulty breathing. Symptoms of asthma include breathlessness, wheezing, insomnia, dry cough, and tightness in the chest that occur in episodes, ranging from mild to severe. A severe attack causes sweating, rapid heartbeat, and extreme gasping for breath. An episode may last from a few minutes to a day. It may be followed by a second or recurring attack that may last for several days or weeks and can be more severe. Asthma is caused by allergies, aspirin products, sulfites, and heredity.

Statistics

Blacks ages five to thirty-four are three to five times more likely than Whites to die from asthma. African American children are particularly susceptible: the hospitalization rate for Black children is two to three times higher than for White children.

Treatments

ACUPRESSURE
Place your fists on your chest with your thumbs pointing upward. Place your thumbs on the muscles that run below your collarbone; gently feel for a sensitive spot. Press firmly and breathe deeply for two minutes. Or reach over your left shoulder with your right hand and press firmly on the part of your back in between your left shoulder blade and spine. Take five breaths and repeat on the right side.

AROMATHERAPY
Try infusions of chamomile, hyssop, or lavender, or use them in hand and foot baths.

CHINESE MEDICINE
Try bitter almond seed or ephedra (**Don't use if you have high blood pressure or heart disease**) for wheezing. To prepare ephedra as a tea: blend 5 grams ephedra, 4 grams cinnamon sticks, 1½ grams licorice, and 5 grams apricot seed. Steep in cold water, then boil. Practitioners also use acupuncture to treat the liver, kidneys, and spleen.

HERBAL REMEDIES
There are many herbal recipes to treat asthma: Add 1 teaspoon of shredded elecampane root to 1 cup cold water. Let stand for ten hours. Strain and heat. Drink hot three times a day. Try aniseed (1 teaspoon crushed seeds to a cup of hot water); chamomile (2 to 3 cups of tea a day); chili (as a tincture, 5 drops three times a day in a glass of water, juice, or herbal tea;) garlic (simmer 1 teaspoon finely chopped garlic, 1 teaspoon finely chopped gin-

gerroot, 2 teaspoons seedless raisins, 1 to 2 tablespoons lemon juice for 15 minutes in 1 cup of water); *Ginkgo biloba* (20 drops three times a day or as a tablet or capsule, see label for dosage); horseradish (as a root, ½ teaspoon grated with food or as a tablet, two after each meal for one to two days, then one after each meal or according to dosage on label); reishi (one to two mushrooms a day or as a tablet, see label for dosage). Put 1 teaspoon apple cider vinegar in warm water and sip slowly. Ginger, green tea, and turmeric also work.

HOMEOPATHY

If your asthma brings on dry wheezing, consider Arsenicum Album 30C (Arsenious Acid). Some cases of asthma have symptoms that may be worse under different conditions, and at different times of the day. Here are some suggestions:

- Natrum Sulphuricum 6C (Sulphate of Sodium)—if worse in evening.

- Aconite 6C (Monkshood)—with dry cough or shortness of breath

MASSAGE

A European-style or shiatsu massage can be helpful in alleviating symptoms.

MIND-BODY

Asthmatics can greatly benefit from calming activities such as yoga, swimming, or hypnosis, which improve breathing and help you relax.

NUTRITION/DIET

If you can, avoid these potential food allergens: meat, citrus fruits, coffee, tea, chocolate, milk, eggs, nuts, seafood; processed foods and food additives such as monosodium glutamate (MSG), and yellow food coloring (Tartrazine). Follow a strict vegetarian diet. Also, take 100 milligrams per day of vitamin B_6 (also found in wheat germ, brewer's yeast, poultry, fish, cooked, dried beans and peas) and 400 to 600 milligrams per day of magnesium.

REFLEXOLOGY

Massage the area between the big toe and second toe on both of your feet. Massage the top of your foot, spreading your toes apart and loosening toe ligaments.

Prevention

Don't smoke if you have asthma (or even if you don't). Cover your mouth and nose in cold weather. Remove potential allergens (which can include pet hair, dust, cockroaches, dust mites in bed linens) from your home and keep it well ventilated. Avoid aspirin and nonsteroidal anti-inflammatory drugs (NSAIDs) that increase your chances of having asthma. Also avoid foods and drinks with high amounts of sulfites (beer, wine, grape and lemon juice, instant tea, white vinegar, dried fruits and canned vegetables).

Bladder Problems

If you've ever experienced the pain of a bladder infection, you'll want to read on to learn how to prevent and treat them. A bladder infection, or urinary tract infection (UTI) is a bacterial infection of the bladder and/or urinary tract. Symptoms include pain or burning during urination; a frequent urge to urinate, or blood in urine; fever; and back and groin pain. If left untreated, a urinary tract infection can spread to the kidneys, causing a serious infection. Anyone can get it, but women seem to be more prone, perhaps because the outside opening of the urethra and vagina are close to the anus, making it easy for bacteria to travel from one area to the other, and because outside bacteria travel easily to the bladder and urinary tract via a woman's urethra, which is only 1 inch long (a man's measures 8 inches). Sexual intercourse can cause bladder infections in women; they are also common during pregnancy.

Incontinence is the inability to control urination due to injury, disease, or weakness of the muscles controlling the bladder. In men, incontinence may also signal prostate problems. Symptoms include leaking urine when coughing, lifting, or laughing. In women, it may occur after childbirth as a result of weakened pelvic floor muscles.

Irritable bladder is the sudden uncontrollable urge to urinate resulting from a bladder infection, bladder stones, or an obstructed flow of urine by an enlarged prostate gland.

Statistics

By age forty, about one-third of all women have experienced at least one UTI. Up to 20 million Americans of all races suffer from incontinence. Seventy-five percent of these are women, and most are elderly.

Treatments

AROMATHERAPY

For UTIs, add 2 drops each of essential oil of juniper berry, eucalyptus, chamomile, parsley, or sandalwood to a warm bath, or massage 5 drops of any of these and 1 ounce vegetable oil over lower back, abdomen, stomach and hips every day. Sit for ten minutes to relieve symptoms. DO NOT USE IF PREGNANT.

CHINESE MEDICINE

For incontinence, practitioners suggest drinking golden lock tea as needed. For UTIs, drink gentian root tea as needed.

CHIROPRACTIC

A practitioner can adjust bones and joints around your pelvis to strengthen bladder muscles and keep urinary tract infections from coming back.

FOLK REMEDIES

For urinary tract infections, drink cranberry juice to acidify urine, preventing bacteria from growing and attaching to wall of bladder. Drink two to four glasses a day.

HERBAL REMEDIES

Holistic practitioners offer the following array of options for you to try: For UTIs, parsley (added to salads and cooked foods) and dandelion leaves (eaten raw in salads) are diuretics (help excrete water and clear infection). Bearberry leaves act as an antiseptic and diuretic. Soak ½ cup of leaves in 2 quarts of cold water for twelve to twenty-four hours. Strain. Drink 1 cup tea up to six times a day.

HOMEOPATHY

If your bladder is irritated and you have the urge to urinate and nothing comes out, Nux Vomica 6C (Poison Nut) is helpful. If you experience pain that is relieved once you urinate, Equisetum 6C (Scouring Rush) will be most effective. When it is actually painful to urinate, Cantharis 6C (Spanish Fly) offers relief. If the pain is felt at the end of urination, Sarsaparilla 6C (Smilax) is the best remedy. Try Apis 6C (Honeybee) if the pain when urinating has a stinging sensation.

Some people have uncontrollable urination after sneezing, laughing or coughing. Causticum 6C (chalk) is recommended in these cases. If urination is uncontrollable when lying down, use Pulsatilla 6C (windflower).

For UTIs, if urination feels violently painful: take Cantharis 6C as a liquid or tablet (see label for dosage); for burning pain at end of urination: take Sarsaparilla 6C as a liquid (see label for dosage); if you have stinging pains that feel better after cold baths: take Apis 6C as a liquid or tablet (see label for dosage); if urination is violently painful, or there is blood in the urine: take Mercurius corrosivus 6C (mercury compound) as a liquid or tablet (see label for dosage) and berberis mother tincture (see label for dosage).

MIND-BODY

For UTIs, it's important to get plenty of rest and take it easy! Try this exercise for irritable bladder and incontinence: squeeze and release your pelvic muscles (as though you're trying to stop the urine flow) when not urinating. This strengthens the pubococcygeus muscle that controls urination. Start with just a few contractions, but do at least five, ten times a day, gradually building up to ten contractions ten times a day or more. Do it while sitting, lying, standing, cooking, or watching television. Once or twice a week, check your progress by stopping the flow while you urinate. After six to eight weeks of exercise, you should find it easier to stop the flow. Also for incontinence, lose any extra pounds—they put pressure on the muscles controlling the bladder.

NUTRITION AND DIET

For UTIs, you should drink at least 8 ounces of water every hour during the first twenty-four hours to flush out bacteria and dilute urine. If you have an irritable bladder, drink at least 2 quarts of water a day. For UTIs, try to avoid alcohol and caffeine in tea, coffee, and soda (it stimulates the kidneys and makes your bladder fill faster, causing painful urination). You need to bulk up on fiber (fruits and vegetables) if you are incontinent.

Other ideas for coping with urinary tract infections: build up your immune system to fight infection by eating lots of raw and lightly cooked vegetables, whole-grain cereals, and low-fat protein. Try to drink lots of water—at least eight glasses a day. Include vitamin A (found in liver, egg yolk, butter/margarine, cheese, cod liver oil) in your diet to help build healthy mucous membranes. If given antibiotics for infection, eat lots of live, unsweetened yogurt with lactobacillus acidophilus—at least one small container a day, for at least one month.

Prevention

For women: Drink eight to ten, 8-ounce glasses of water a day to dilute your urine. Keep your vaginal and anal areas clean; wipe from front to back. Don't wear tight-fitting clothing (it traps heat and promotes bacterial growth). Wear cotton underwear (air circulates better). Be sure to empty your bladder after intercourse and try to avoid intercourse during menstruation. Change tampons and sanitary napkins frequently. And don't hold it in—urinate when you get the urge. For incontinence, follow the same advice as above. Also avoid scented soaps, talc, and deodorants in your genital area. Go to the toilet only when your bladder is full. Drink at least 2 quarts of any liquid a day.

 Testimonial

Suzanne Nesbitt (not her real name), twenty-six, suffers from UTIs. She believes it's because she doesn't "go" when she feels the urge. As a teacher with a regimented schedule, she needs to fit in bathroom breaks whenever she can get away from the classroom—which means only one to two per day for her. "You put yourself on the clock for going to the bathroom!" she says. What works to relieve Suzanne's symptoms? Pure cranberry juice with no sugar, diluted with water. "I drink it by the quart and it works."

Bowel Problems

It seems as though every other television commercial has something to do with your digestive system, such as laxatives, antacids, and antidiarrheal drugs. If you suffer from bowel problems, perhaps you can find relief from one of the alternative treatments below.

Constipation, which is very common, includes these symptoms: irregular, infrequent, dry, or difficult bowel movements. It is caused by stress, lack of exercise, or not taking in enough fiber or fluids.

If you have diarrhea, which is also very common, you experience urgent and watery stools. It is caused by a virus, food sensitivities (such as lactose, which is a sugar found in milk), bacteria, prescription antibiotics, using artificial sweeteners, or high doses of vitamin C.

Indigestion sufferers have mild nausea, gas, and bloating. It is caused by fatty or fried foods, spicy or highly acidic foods, eating too much food or eating too fast, and stress.

Colitis (Crohn's disease, ulcerative colitis) is an inflammation of the large intestine with diarrhea, severe abdominal pain, fever, diarrhea, fatigue, sore joints, or loss of appetite. Ulcerative colitis is a chronic disease where the colon develops tiny ulcers and inflammations that flare up, causing painful, bloody stools. Crohn's disease is a chronic condition where the gastrointestinal tract becomes inflamed and weak, causing problems with digestion. The cause of each is unknown, but symptoms can occur after taking antibiotics such as penicillin, amoxicillin, or tetracycline and Crohn's disease may be the result of the immune system attacking part of the intestine.

Irritable bowel syndrome (IBS) includes symptoms of crampy pain, gassiness, bloating, alternating diarrhea and constipation, hard stools resulting from stress or improper functioning of the large intestine. It occurs when the contractions that allow the intestines to move food through the intestinal tract become unco-ordinated and digestion is disrupted. The cause is unknown, but stress, antibiotics and some medications, a fatty diet, food sensitiv-ities, overeating, or smoking may bring it about.

Statistics

Approximately 50 million Americans suffer from constipation oc-casionally or regularly. Inflammatory bowel syndrome affects at least 10 to 15 percent of all American adults; Blacks are just as likely as Whites to have it. Inflammatory bowel disease affects about 2 million Americans; Whites are five times more likely than Blacks to have it, and females more likely than males.

Treatments

ACUPRESSURE

Bowel problems are related to large intestine flow, which cor-responds to the arm, from the index finger up to the shoulder and part of the face. If you have a blockage in the intestine and press along the inner elbow, that area will probably be tender. Also, press inward with your index finger on the abdominal area about three finger-widths below the navel, then inhale slowly and deeply, and exhale. This will relieve abdominal pain. This also works: using the thumb and index finger of your right hand, squeeze the area between the thumb and index finger of your left hand for one minute. Repeat on the right hand. **Do not do this if you're pregnant.**

ACUPUNCTURE

In acupuncture, the spleen encompasses the digestive process. So any enzyme related to the digestive tract is called spleen energy. For IBS, a practitioner may insert needles along the liver, spleen, and kidney meridians. For diarrhea, a practitioner may insert nee-dles near the navel and left knee.

AROMATHERAPY/MASSAGE

For indigestion, try the following technique. Either lying or sitting, massage your abdomen in a clockwise direction with 1 drop essential oil of peppermint or ginger.

For IBS, massage your abdomen gently with a mixture of 3 drops of essential oil of peppermint, 3 drops essential oil of black pepper, and 4 teaspoons carrier oil or lotion. Put one hand on top of the other and gently knead your stomach, using small, circular motions. Start at the right bottom corner moving upward to the right of your lower limbs, down to the left bottom corner, and back across to the right.

If you have colitis (Crohn's disease), use essential oil of lavender in a diffuser, in a bath, or through steam inhalation to relieve stress. Also, a few drops of Roman or German chamomile in warm water dipped in a towel can be made into a compress and placed on the abdomen.

COLON HYDROTHERAPY

According to Ayurvedic medicine, if you have three meals a day, you should eliminate at least three times a day. Your colon should be like an empty trash bag, but months and years of residual waste can cause toxicity. Visit a certified colon hydrotherapist to clean out your colon, and follow a high-fiber diet to increase the bulk passing through the colon.

FOLK REMEDIES

To settle your stomach, eat a grated apple that has turned brown. For diarrhea, drink flat ginger ale, chicken broth, and weak (nonherbal) tea.

HERBAL REMEDIES

There are numerous herbal remedies for bowel problems. The following are a few suggestions from holistic practitioners:

For constipation: drink a goldenseal infusion. Add 2 teaspoons dried root goldenseal to 1 cup boiling water. Steep for fifteen minutes. You also might want to try these stimulants for constipation: cascara sagrada bark, buckthorn bark, senna, or *Aloe vera* gel capsules. Take ½ teaspoon each per dosage. **Do not take if breast-feeding.** For diarrhea: drink peppermint, blackberry root, wood betony, raspberry, or blueberry chamomile tea. Add 1 to 2 teaspoons of leaves to 1 cup boiling water. Steep ten to fifteen minutes (twenty minutes for blackberry root). For indigestion, try strong, hot peppermint tea or chamomile tea, crushed caraway, fennel, or anise teas. For IBS, a peppermint infusion relieves spasms and gas: add 1 teaspoon dried herb to 1 cup boiling water. Infuse for ten minutes. For colitis (Crohn's disease, ulcerative colitis), take garlic or use in cooking.

HOMEOPATHY

There are a number of conditions that cause bowel disorders. Here is a list of good and effective homeopathic remedies:

- Nux Vomica 6C (Poison Nut)—urge for bowel movement with no result along with spasms.

- Cina 6C (Worm-Seed)—colic; diarrhea; gas.

- Arsenicum 6C (Arsenious Acid)—burning diarrhea with chills.

- Aloe 6C (Socotrine Aloe)—burning rectum and loose stools.

- Podophyllum 6C (May Apple)—stomach cramps with green stools.

MIND-BODY

Exercise stimulates bowel movements, so get moving with an activity you enjoy. You can alleviate stress, a trigger of many bowel problems, through meditation or stress-reduction techniques. For colitis, strengthen abdominal muscles with sit-ups or curl downs (sit on floor with knees bent, lean back halfway to floor with back rounded, count to two, curl back up). For Crohn's disease, avoid stress or relieve it with exercise, meditation, and/ or massage.

NUTRITION AND DIET

For constipation, eat fresh fruit, especially in the morning, to cleanse the colon, or try dried prunes, apricots, figs, or a large glass of prune juice (they all contain a natural laxative). Make sure to eat plenty of fresh vegetables, beans, and fiber (at least 30 grams a day of either whole-grain bread, pasta, brown rice, miller's bran, or oatmeal). Try to drink at least eight glasses of water a day— a warm glass of water when you wake up sometimes helps get things "moving."

For diarrhea, make sure the condition isn't caused by a food allergy, such as to milk. To avoid dehydration, add 1 teaspoon salt and 1 tablespoon sugar to 1 quart boiled water and 1 pint orange or lemon juice. Drink 1 pint every hour until symptoms go away. Eating live yogurt with *Lactobacillus acidophilus* restores the balance of good bacteria in the digestive tract. Also, drink lots of clear fluids and diluted juices.

For indigestion, eat small, regular meals. What's the rush? Eat slowly and chew your food completely. Make sure your diet includes lots of vegetables, bread, brown rice, and whole-grain pasta instead of refined carbohydrates. Avoid fried foods and sauces— broil or grill instead.

For IBS, follow the treatment for constipation and diarrhea. Because IBS is often linked to lactose intolerance, try avoiding all dairy products for two weeks and see if symptoms improve. Keep a diary to find out possible food triggers; also note how you felt after eating. Try to eat lots of unsweetened live yogurt with *Lactobacillus acidophilus.*

For Crohn's disease, increase vitamin A, beta-carotene, and vitamin D. Take vitamin B complex once a day.

REFLEXOLOGY

For indigestion, massage the area above the middle of the arch on the soles of your feet.

Prevention

You should bulk up on fiber and drink plenty of fluids every day. Exercise! Avoid sorbitol and mannitol (artificial sweeteners that can cause diarrhea). For indigestion, avoid spicy or rich foods; drink plenty of water between meals, although not much during; and avoid going to bed on a full stomach. For Crohn's disease, avoid stress.

Consider food intolerances that might make your system sluggish such as bread, nuts, eggs, fish, and milk. Many adults, including a significant number of African Americans, are lactose-intolerant, which can cause bloating, gas, cramping, and diarrhea.

Breast Problems

For women, there are changes that occur in their breasts that are associated with puberty, their menstrual cycle, pregnancy, and age. These problems may include tenderness, pain, lumps, or other noncancerous conditions in one or both breasts. Breast pain can be caused by normal swelling or hormonal changes during the menstrual cycle, infection, injury, growth, or diet. Lumps, which come in the form of cysts, adenomas, and papillomas, are attributed to normal breast changes related to hormonal shifts immediately before or during the menstrual cycle (due to increases in estrogen and progesterone, or more fluid in the breasts). Other causes include injury, infection, diet, and sometimes cancer (for information on breast cancer, see page 221). Fibrocystic breast disease is a condition that causes painful, lumpy, swollen, tender breasts. It is critical for all women to do monthly breast self-examinations and on discovery of a lump, to contact a physician immediately.

Statistics
Sixty percent of all women suffer from fibrocystic breast disease.

Treatments

AROMATHERAPY
For pain relief, use 6 to 8 drops essential oil of geranium in a hot bath. Or try this: Massage your breasts with a mixture of 15 drops essential oil of geranium in 3 tablespoons bland carrier oil or lotion.

AYURVEDIC MEDICINE
For fibrocystic disease, mix 1 teaspoon turmeric and 1 teaspoon warm castor oil, apply to breasts where cysts are, and cover with cloth (turmeric does stain your clothes) before going to bed.

HERBAL REMEDIES
Take evening primrose oil supplements (500 milligrams two or three times a day) for breast lumps. For breast tenderness, eat lots of chopped fresh parsley to help your body expel excess water.

HOMEOPATHY
The homeopathic remedy Scrophularia Nodosa 6C (Knotted Figwood) has a specific use for breast tumors. It is usually administered professionally by a homeopath. Don't expect to find it over-the-counter at your local health food store.

Many nursing mothers experience some common problems as a result of breast-feeding. With pain that starts in the nipple and radiates all over the body, or heavy breasts with hard lumps, try Phytolacca 6X or 12C (Poke Root).

Pulsatilla 12C (windFlower) given immediately upon stopping nursing will often help to dry up the milk supply. On the other hand, Calcarea Carbonica 6C (Carbonate of Lime) may help to increase milk supply.

Remember the remedies will not hurt the baby.

For many women, the formation of cysts throughout the breasts, with pain and tenderness, caused either by diet or hormonal imbalances can be a real problem. In these cases, Bryonia 30C makes the condition better.

HYDROTHERAPY

For pain relief, apply a hot, moist compress to your breasts for three to five minutes when you take a shower followed by sponging your breasts with cool water.

MASSAGE

Get a professional massage to help increase the circulation to and from the lymph nodes and prevent a buildup of toxins in your body.

MIND/BODY

If you're overweight, shed that girth. Exercise to stimulate blood circulation to your breasts, which helps to clear toxins. You can reduce stress with meditation and by getting enough sleep.

NUTRITION AND DIET

For breast lumps, increase your intake of vitamin A, B-complex vitamins, beta-carotene, and fiber. Take vitamin E (400 to 1200 IU per day) to help absorb vitamin A. Take selenium (found in whole wheat, rice, oatmeal, poultry, low-fat dairy products, lean meats, organ meats, fish, and seafood) or as a supplement (no more than 150 micrograms a day). Cut back on fat and caffeine. For breast tenderness, reduce salt, alcohol, and coffee. Eat plenty of fruits and vegetables, and low-fat protein.

Prevention

Examine your breasts once a month; and after your period, check for lumps or other changes. Follow the diet as described above. Try wearing a support bra to lessen discomfort.

Cancer

In this day and age, we have all become familiar with "the big C," which includes more than 100 diseases affecting practically every organ and limb in our bodies. Cancer is the unrestricted growth of cells in an organ or tissues that interfere with the normal functioning of the body. According to physicians, genes normally control the division of cells, which occurs to replace cells that die. When genes malfunction, cells can grow uncontrolled, causing harmless (benign) tumors or dangerous (malignant) tumors. Cells from malignant tumors can spread to nearby tissues or throughout the body, where they cause other tumors.

The most common sites of cancer include the breasts, lungs, intestines, prostate, colon, lymphatic system, stomach, skin, blood (leukemia), and pancreas. Cancer also occurs in the bones and muscles (sarcoma), but this is rare. Classic signs and symptoms include a sore that doesn't heal within three weeks; a mole on the skin that itches, bleeds, or grows; a lump or swelling beneath the skin; recurring indigestion or difficulty swallowing; hoarseness that lasts longer than one week; a persistent cough or coughing up blood; a change in bowel or bladder habits; blood in urine or stools; and vaginal bleeding after your regular period or after menopause. The causes: viruses (such as hepatitis B virus, which causes liver cancer); chemicals (particularly tobacco, which causes cancer of the lung, tongue, larynx, cervix, and bladder); heredity; diet (excessive alcohol, fat, smoked foods); and radiation (x-rays, sunlight, nuclear waste). Cancer is rare among people in their twenties but risk doubles between ages thirty and forty and doubles again with each passing decade.

Statistics

Breast cancer is the leading cause of cancer death among Black women. The five-year survival rate for Blacks is 43 percent compared with 90 percent for White women. Black men have the highest incidence of prostate cancer in the world. African Americans as a whole are more likely than Whites to have their cancer diagnosed at a later stage, and are less likely to receive advanced treatment.

Treatments

ACUPUNCTURE

Although it is not documented to arrest cancer, acupuncture is known to relieve pain and increase strength.

HERBAL REMEDIES

Catharanthus roseus (take as a liquid or tablet) contains two naturally occurring chemicals that appear in anticancer pharmaceuticals. Drugs derived from May apple roots (take as a liquid or tablet) are used to treat lymphomas, lung cancer, and leukemia. Garlic (take as a fresh clove or tablet) may contain anticancer compounds that help stimulate the immune system and halt growth of cancer cells. Black tea, green tea, and oolong tea (consult a naturopath for dosage) contain catechins, which may block development of some cancers. Horsetail (taken as a dried or fresh herb, capsule, or tincture) may prevent hair loss after chemotherapy. Ginger (taken as a fresh or dried root, extract, tablet, capsule, or tea) may reduce nausea from chemotherapy or radiation. Consult a naturopath for additional information.

HOMEOPATHY

Nux vomica and phosphorus may help alleviate nausea from chemotherapy.

MASSAGE

Massage does not arrest cancer, but promotes relaxation, eases pain, and releases emotions.

MIND-BODY

Try meditation, breathing exercises, guided imagery, progressive muscle relaxation, hypnotherapy, biofeedback, and visualization to relieve discomfort (pain, nausea, or vomiting from treatment), stress, anxiety, and depression. Exercise helps control fatigue, muscle tension, anxiety, so you might try yoga, walking, or swimming. Immerse yourself in activities you enjoy, whether it's shopping with a friend or listening to music. And don't discount counseling, whether alone or in a group, as a means of support from others who know what you're going through.

NUTRITION AND DIET

Eat plenty of fresh organic fruits and vegetables and whole-grain cereals. Include lean meats and low-fat seafood. You should avoid processed foods, smoked or cured meat, food additives, and sugar, and reduce animal fat and alcohol. Get plenty of vitamins A, C, E, B_6, selenium, magnesium, folic acid, and zinc.

REFLEXOLOGY

Reflexology does not arrest cancer, but promotes relaxation, eases pain, and releases emotions.

Prevention

Don't smoke; avoid prolonged exposure to sunlight without a sunblock; eat a fiber-rich diet; reduce fat, meat, sugar, alcohol. Eat lots of beta-carotene-rich foods (such as carrots, squash or melons), vitamin C, selenium (found in seafood, brewer's yeast, whole-grain cereals), and vitamin E (found in nuts, wheat germ, apples, broccoli). Avoid food additives, nitrates, or contaminated or moldy foods. Keep your weight and stress under control. Get plenty of regular exercise. Limit exposure to carcinogenic chemicals at work and home (pesticides, aerosol cleaning products, or paint). Plan to get screened for breast, cervical, intestinal, and prostate cancer during your annual checkup. Ladies, examine your breasts monthly.

Medical Research is Proving What Black Folks Have Always Known: Prayer Heals

"He's the doctor who never lost a case." You can hear that affirmation in deacons' prayers in just about any Black church in America. And there are miraculous testimonies given in churches all across the world from people who say they prayed their cancer into remission or threw away their high blood pressure medicine, replacing it with meditation and spiritual focusing.

Until lately, such exercises of prayer and faith have been written off as one-in-a-million phenomena, rather than an actual method of healing that could help cure disease. But with an increasing number of people claiming prayer has healed their diseases—or at the very least made life a little less stressful while dealing with disease and discomfort—the scientific and medical communities are beginning to take note.

There are hundreds of studies published in the medical literature since the nineteenth century in which spiritual or religious practices have been statistically proven to have positive health outcomes for everything from cardiovascular disease, hypertension, stroke, and nearly every type of cancer to something as simple as the common cold.

But more recently, research has begun to more carefully quantify the connection between health and spirituality. In the past few years, major studies have shown that people who attend church are less likely to have stress-related health problems and are more likely to survive surgery. Church-going smokers were less likely to have high blood pressure than nonchurch goers.

Prestigious bastions of medical science such as Harvard, Georgetown, and Johns Hopkins Universities have begun to include courses dealing with religion and medicine. This year Morehouse School of Medicine in Atlanta, Georgia, became one of only eight schools—and the only historically Black medical school—in the nation to offer a spirituality course to its medical candidates. And respected medical researchers from Massachusetts to California have established institutes to further the research in the field.

Look at the work of Larry Dossey, M.D., a leader in the field and author of *Healing Words: The Power of Prayer and the Practice of Medicine* (Harper Collins, 1994). Dossey reports in his book on a 1988 study conducted at San Francisco General Medical Center in which one group of randomly assigned coronary care patients was prayed for, while another group was not. The people who did the praying were given only the patients' first names and their general conditions, but were not told what to pray for specifically, or how to pray. Each patient in the experiment had between three and seven people praying for him or her. The results found that patients who were prayed for were five times less likely to require antibiotics and three times less likely to develop cardiopulmonary arrest. And fewer of them died than in the group not prayed for.

"If the technique being studied had been a new drug or a surgical procedure instead of prayer," according to Dr.

Dossey, "it would almost certainly have been heralded as some sort of breakthrough."

But while prayer has yet to be heralded as such, some doctors regularly incorporate it into their practice. Deborah McGregor, M.D., whose Philadelphia, Pennsylvania, internal medicine practice specializes in Ayurvedic and Chinese medicine, employs two spiritualists to regularly pray for patients and encourages patients to pray for each other.

"We hold telephone ministries with our patients and take names of people who want special prayer," she explains. "Our nursing home patients also pray regularly for 'all of Dr. McGregor's patients,' and they ask regularly how so-and-so is doing."

Scientific studies aside, Dr. McGregor has seen firsthand that praying can make a difference. "I allow my patients to be in a prayerful and spiritual state when I treat them, and I let them know that I have a personal connection with God through my faith that he will provide the best way for me to treat them."

Her efforts are probably appreciated. Gallup Polls show that 40 percent of the population want their doctors to pray with them.

Valencia Clay, M.D., assistant professor at the Morehouse School of Medicine, where she teaches the school's first course on spirituality, has also used prayer while working with patients.

"I pray for different reasons, but mostly I pray for God to help me with difficult diagnoses," she says. And she's found that of the patients she sees, those who maintain a sense of faith do far better than those who have given up. "Even terminal cases realize it's not the end of life, but in a sense it's a beginning."

While prayer can work to comfort the minds of those in pain and facilitate transition from life to death in the case of some terminal illnesses, there are many cases of people eradicating serious conditions, leaving doctors baffled.

"Prayer has to do with a person's belief system and just how far they want to take it," says Roxbury, Massachusetts, massage therapist and energy-field healer Bonita Buchanan-Jones. "For some, their prayer and faith is so strong, an actual healing takes place; while for others, making a peaceful transition is enough, and that's okay."

The latter was the case for one of Dr. McGregor's patients who was dying of cancer. "All she wanted to do was hold on until her son could get to the hospital," Dr. McGregor recalls. "That's what we prayed for. As soon as her son, who was stationed on a ship, got there, she perked up and told him what she needed to tell him. She was then able to make her transition at peace." She died as soon as he left the hospital.

Dr. Barbara L. King, metaphysical author and minister at Hillside Chapel and Truth Center in Atlanta, Georgia, grew up with a thyroid condition that caused a lump in her throat. She went without treatment for most of her adult life, although she noticed that the lump would shrink or swell, depending on her emotional state. "I was resistant to surgery, so I wore high collars and scarves to try to hide the problem, and said I was going to pray this thing out of here."

After seeking medical advice, however, her doctor recommended an operation because of the size of the swelling and because it was beginning to press against her windpipe, making it a wonder that she had been able to talk. "Throughout the ordeal, I was conditioning my thoughts to God thoughts," she says. She grew stronger in her spiritual practices and continued to pray daily. "I never gave up on God, and I never had a fear thought."

Just before the operation, Dr. King, two friends, and her doctor prayed that the surgeon might be able to perform the surgery without any problems.

"The surgeon made the incision and went in with his various instruments and got ready to cut around the lump, but he didn't have to cut anything," she says. "The thing popped out on its own. The healing was always going on. They call it a miracle; I call it God."

Dr. King is a firm believer that: "You don't have to just live with anything. The first step in healing is to condition your mind to God thoughts; the second step is to surrender. Get your human emotions out of the way, sit back, and everything will fall into place."

Who you call on when you pray for healing doesn't seem to make a difference, studies suggest. Whether it's Allah, Buddha, or Jesus Christ, healing seems to be facilitated more by a commitment to any faith rather than a specific belief, according to Dr. Dossey.

For those who want to incorporate prayer into their healing strategy, the major question isn't "to whom?" but "for what?" Should you pray specifically to get rid of an illness or pray a nondirected prayer like "Thy will be done"?

Although some say that when you pray, you should be specific, according to Dr. Dossey's research, nondirected prayer—asking for guidance or giving thanks—seems to work better than asking, "God, kill my cancer."

In fact, prayer isn't something you do, according to Dossey's theories, it's something you are. Being prayerful brings about a willingness to accept healing when it comes your way.

"Prayer is every thought you think, every word you speak and every action you take," says best-selling author and Yoruba priestess Iyanla Vanzant.

For that reason, she believes it is always important to pray in the affirmative, acknowledging that what you ask for already exists and is just waiting to manifest. "Whatever you believe will determine the efficacy of your prayer. If you believe in cancer, pain, and suffering, that's what you'll get," she says.

She also advises that prayer (talking to God) always be followed by meditation (listening to God). "What we do is pray and then get busy—getting all in the middle of things, blocking our healing—when what we should do is get still. Give the universe a chance to respond to our needs."

"Prayer and meditation are a part of the same healing continuum. Both represent a personal, private communion with spirit," says Dr. McGregor.

Knowing how to incorporate faith and spirituality when faced with a challenging disease or ailment can be difficult to understand.

"Sometimes there may be a misunderstanding about medicine and religion on the patient's part," says Morehouse School of Medicine's Dr. Clay. "They may believe it's a lack of faith to be treated by a doctor, but if you talk with them and help them understand that God gives doctors knowledge to help people heal, you can clear up any misunderstanding."

One of the aims of Dr. Clay's course at Morehouse is to teach future doctors to understand and respect a patient's beliefs.

Although Dr. King maintained herself in a prayerful state of mind throughout her ordeal, she is quick to warn against thinking that prayer by itself is enough.

"It takes prayer and action," explains Dr. King, who also followed a strict herbal and nutritional program for about a year prior to the surgery. "You have to follow through with an act of faith."

That may mean seeing your doctor for regular check-ups, changing your diet, starting an exercise program—affirmative activities that can be part of your personal healing program. Other than Christian Scientists, who don't believe in medical intervention at all, even the most avowed spiritualist wouldn't turn away good health care.

"Prayer isn't about begging God to help you. He's already

helped you. His work is done. Now it's up to you to accept the responsibility for your healing," Vanzant says.

Cholesterol Problems

While there are some fatty foods that are simply hard to resist—bacon, burgers, or french fries, for example—eventually, they take a toll on our bodies. Cholesterol (a yellow, waxy fat) is essential for health, but only in small does. It's an important ingredient of your cell membranes, some hormones, and vitamin D. That's why your body makes cholesterol in addition to what you may get from bacon and burgers. But too much cholesterol is bad news. If your blood cholesterol level maxes out, cholesterol can build up on your artery walls, clogging them and restricting blood flow. This leads to high blood pressure, heart attack, stroke, or angina. There are two types of cholesterol in your bloodstream: high-density lipoprotein (HDL)—good cholesterol—and low-density lipoprotein (LDL)—the bad stuff. You want high levels of HDL and low levels of LDL and a low total cholesterol level overall. High cholesterol runs in some families, especially if diabetes or obesity is common.

Statistics
Obesity increases the risk of high cholesterol levels. Approximately 36 percent of all Black women are overweight compared with 21 percent of White women. And 60 percent of middle-aged Black women are notably overweight compared with 28 percent of middle-aged White women.

Treatments

AYURVEDIC MEDICINE
Practitioners use Malabar tamarind (Brindall berry), an Indian fruit, for obesity. It may also help reduce cholesterol levels.

CHINESE MEDICINE
Acupuncture together with the herb polygonum can treat high cholesterol.

HERBAL REMEDIES
Try drinking Chinese green tea or oolong tea instead of coffee, which raises cholesterol levels. Spirulina, a protein-rich alga, reduces total cholesterol and LDL levels, plus it's got chlorophyll, amino acids, vitamins, and minerals. It's available in tablets or powder form at natural food stores. The Indian remedy gugulipid (from the mukul myrrh tree) helps control cholesterol levels. Consult a naturopath for dosage. Also good for lowering cholesterol are alfalfa (taken as a tea, tincture, capsule, dried leaves, powdered extract, or sprouts); turmeric (taken as a powdered root, capsule, liquid extract); Asian ginseng (taken as fresh, dried, or freeze-dried root, root powder, capsule, tablet, prepared tea, rock candy); fenugreek (taken as seeds, capsule, or tincture), and phytosterols (see a naturopath for dosage).

MIND-BODY
The more overweight you are, the more cholesterol your body produces, so keep your weight in check by getting two-thirds of your calories from fruits, vegetables, cereals, and whole grains, and one-third of your calories from meat and dairy products. To raise your HDL (good cholesterol) levels, lower your LDL levels, and decrease build-up of any fatty deposits that may be lurking in your arteries, exercise aerobically thirty minutes or more three times a week—jogging, swimming, or brisk walking are all good options.

Meditation, guided imagery, yoga, biofeedback, massage, or simple relaxation can lower total cholesterol levels by alleviating stress. Find a quiet place; sit on a firm surface; and close your eyes. Allow your breathing to slow. Begin to feel aware of how your body feels. Relax each part of your body from head to toe, one by one. Do it for ten minutes.

NUTRITION AND DIET

When you bake, reduce fat by using one-third to one-half of the called-for olive, canola, or peanut oil. Make up the difference by adding water. Try low-fat or nonfat frozen yogurt, ice cream, or luncheon meat. (They really do taste good!) Substitute low-fat or nonfat plain yogurt for sour cream as a topping, and herbs and spices for butter or margarine. Cut down on eggs (don't eat more than three a week), and avoid the yolk, which has all the cholesterol, or try cholesterol-free egg substitutes (in your grocer's dairy case) or lower-cholesterol eggs sold in some stores.

Eat lots of poultry (without the skin), and dried peas and beans—all good sources of protein. Go fish: omega-3 fatty acids found in fish oils reduce blood cholesterol and LDL cholesterol, raise HDL cholesterol, and reduce risk of developing cardiovascular disease. Unload your deep-fat fryer at a garage sale. Instead, try baking, broiling, or roasting meat, poultry, and fish. If you must have your cow (and eat it, too), buy as lean and mean a cut as you can find. Drink skim, low-fat, or nonfat milk and other dairy products. Eat a raw onion and two to three garlic cloves a day (or take three garlic capsules, three times a day) to reduce harmful blood fats.

Beta-carotene (found in carrots, broccoli, and cabbage), vitamin C, and vitamin E can raise HDL (good cholesterol) levels. Add to your hot cereal, pancakes, or muffins some oat bran, rice bran, or corn bran (all contain soluble fiber) to lower your serum cholesterol. Soybeans and soy products are also a good source of bran.

The fiber found in fruits (pectin), alfalfa, and cooked, dried beans helps reduce cholesterol levels.

Talk with your doctor before taking these supplements to lower cholesterol: niacin, vitamin C, vitamin E, and calcium.

Take 1 tablespoon a day of flax oil (Inositol hexaminiciati) to reduce high fat levels in blood. If you have diabetes, use pantothine (vitamin B_5). Prevent high cholesterol with a high-fiber diet including carrots, oat fiber, psyllium seeds, omega-3 oils, or fish. Reduce the fat intake in your diet to no more than 30 percent of your daily calories. Eat lots of fruits and vegetables.

Prevention

Your arteries begin collecting fatty deposits at a tender age, so you're never too young to start off right by eating a low-fat, high-fiber diet. Keep a good balance of HDL and LDL by following this diet throughout your life and have your cholesterol checked every one to three years, depending on your age and overall health. Generally, a total blood cholesterol level below 200 mg/dL is good; 200 to 239 is borderline; 240 and above is high. Check food labels for cholesterol and saturated fat that may be hiding behind names like palm oil, coconut oil, egg yolk solids, shortening, hydrogenated oils, lard, or beef fat. Maintain a healthy weight for your height and age, and exercise regularly. Quit smoking.

Common Cold or Flu

Most of us don't make it through the year without suffering through a cold or a bout with the flu. We find ourselves curled up under a blanket sipping chicken soup and downing orange juice by the quart. The common cold is caused by viruses that inflame the mucous membranes lining the nose and throat, bringing on a stuffy, runny nose, sore throat, sneezing, headache, and fatigue. The virus is transmitted by breathing infected droplets from someone else's sneeze or cough, or by touching their (infected) mucous membranes, then yours. Colds usually last three to seven days.

Flu is caused by an influenza virus that brings fever, headache, joint pain, stomach upset, and a stuffy or runny nose. It is transmitted like colds. Aches, pain, and fever usually last two to five days, and fatigue and cough can last for several weeks. Flu can lead to pneumonia and can be fatal for elderly people, very young children, and people with heart or chronic lung disease.

Statistics

Influenza and pneumonia are the eighth leading cause of death among Black males and seventh leading cause of death among Black females.

Treatments

AROMATHERAPY

Essential oil of tea tree and lemon are useful in combating infection. Use 1 drop of each in steam inhalations (add the oil to a basin of steaming water, lean over the basin, covering your head and the basin with a towel, and inhale deeply).

For chest congestion, steam inhalation with 1 to 2 drops of essential oil of eucalyptus or peppermint works wonders. (If you have asthma, put a few drops of the oil on a tissue and inhale instead.)

CHINESE MEDICINE

Astragalus boosts the immune system and increases the production of white blood cells. Use as a tincture or in capsule form.

FOLK REMEDIES

Good old-fashioned chicken soup clears a stuffy nose because it loosens mucus and may boost the immune system. Gargle with salt water (1 teaspoon salt with 8 ounces warm water) three times a day to soothe a sore throat. Rub your chest with mineral oil and Vicks Vapo-Rub salve to relieve congestion. Take castor oil or cod liver oil to help the body "throw off" a cold. The saying, "feed a cold, starve a fever" may apply—eat if you're hungry, but cut back on congestive foods that create a lot of mucus such as milk products, fatty foods, and meat. Add more fresh fruits and vegetables instead.

HERBAL REMEDIES

Echinacea boosts the immune system, lessening the effects of a cold or flu. It cleans your blood and lymph glands, which help circulate infection-fighting antibodies and remove toxic substances. Take one or two capsules twice a day for up to two weeks. Drink as a tea (2 teaspoons echinacea root to 1 cup warm water). **Pregnant or breastfeeding women: use only with your physician's approval.**

Garlic has antiviral and antibacterial properties that kill germs and clear up cold symptoms. In capsules, tablets, cooked, or chewed raw, it can cut the duration of a cold. Take two or three oil-free garlic capsules three times a day, or sip a garlic and onion broth.

Goldenseal contains the natural antibiotic berberine, which helps clear mucous membranes in the nose, mouth, and throat. It stimulates the liver, which helps clear up infections. To soothe a sore throat, gargle cooled goldenseal tea. (Use 1 teaspoon dried, powdered root per cup of boiling water. Steep for ten minutes.) **Pregnant or breastfeeding women and those with high blood pressure, heart disease, diabetes, glaucoma, or a history of stroke should not use.**

Ginger helps relieve nausea and diarrhea caused by the stomach flu. It also clears nasal congestion, reduces fever, and relieves coughs, and helps boost your immune system and kills the flu virus. Try drinking it as a tea by adding a thumb-size piece of fresh ginger and about 2 tablespoons crushed cinnamon stick to a quart of water. Boil twenty minutes; and add lemon and honey if desired.

Peppermint contains menthol, which helps clear head and chest congestion. Tea made from fresh herbs or prepared tea bags can silence a cough. (Combine equal parts of peppermint, elder, and yarrow; steep 1 to 2 teaspoons of it in 1 cup hot water.)

Zinc lozenges can reduce your cold suffering to fewer than five days and alleviate sore throat, stuffy and runny nose, coughing, and sneezing. Take the amount recommended by your physician or pharmacist: it can be toxic in large doses. Boneset infusion relieves the aches, fever, and congestion of the flu. Pour 1 cup of boiling water on 2 teaspoons dried herb, and steep for fifteen minutes.

HOMEOPATHY

To address the symptoms of a cold or flu that include fatigue, tiredness, chills, and aching limbs, you will find Gelsemium 6C (Yellow Jasmine) is good to soothe and calm. If your symptoms reflect more congestion in the head, with a runny nose and irritability, try Nux Vomica 6C (Poison Nut).

MIND-BODY

Get plenty of rest so you can reserve all of your strength for fending off your cold or flu and you won't get sicker. Take a few days off from work if you can, and get more sleep than usual. Wearing yourself out physically compromises your immune system, prolonging your cold. Adopt a positive attitude. Sometimes "thinking" healthy and visualizing a well body can make the difference between a cold lasting a couple of days versus a couple of weeks.

NUTRITION AND DIET

At the first sign of a cold or flu, decrease overall food intake, but eat plenty of fruits, vegetables, soups, and salads. These are alkaline foods that act to neutralize the acidic internal environment that bacteria and viruses love.

Drink plenty of water, tea, and juice—six to eight glasses a day—to replace lost fluids and flush out impurities. Load up on citrus fruits or take vitamin C supplements (between 1,500 and 3,000 milligrams a day) to help reduce coughing, sneezing, and other symptoms. For flu, eat more lean meat, fish, and whole-grain breads and cereals, which contain zinc.

REFLEXOLOGY

Flu is a respiratory condition, so you'll want to contact a qualified reflexologist and ask about having work done on areas that cleanse and drain your body of toxins, via foot and hand systems that control the lymphatic glands, spleen, adrenal gland, and diaphragm.

Prevention

To avoid cold misery, keep your immune system strong. Eat a low-fat, high-fiber diet with lots of whole-grain cereals; green, orange, and yellow vegetables; fruits; fish and poultry; and low-fat dairy products to provide sufficient vitamins and minerals. Add a multivitamin during or after a cold when immunity is low, and a vitamin C supplement twice a day. Eat fewer fatty foods, meats, and milk products.

Quit smoking altogether, or at least while you have a cold— it aggravates an already aggravated sore throat. And it interferes with the body's ability to rid itself of bacteria in the lungs and throat.

Depression

More than just the blues, depression involves insomnia, loss of appetite, or weight loss or gain, either hyperactivity or loss of interest in activity, loss of usual interests, lethargy, difficulty making decisions, either loss of interest in sex or sudden extreme interest in sex, feelings of worthlessness or guilt, crying spells, difficulty concentrating, feelings of self-hate, headaches, backaches, digestive problems, suicidal thoughts or attempts, or overwhelming feelings of anxiety, sadness, or hopelessness. To be classified as clinical depression, at least four symptoms must be present and must last at least two weeks.

The causes of depression vary. Some include the pressure to do it all and have it all, followed by unmet expectations; heredity; postpartum period; premenstrual syndrome; chronic diseases; alcoholism; infectious diseases; medications; seasonal affective disorder; or a stressful life event (death of a loved one, breakup with your mate, loss of a job, etc.). Many depressed people (particularly Black women, many of whom equate depression with weakness or don't believe they have the right to feel as bad as they do) suffer in silence—which only makes depression worse.

Statistics

Nine million American adults suffer from a depressive illness in any six-month period. It is the most common mental disorder in America, and affects twice as many women as men. Black women have 42 percent higher rates of depression than White women.

Treatments

AROMATHERAPY

Try breathing essential oils of basil, clary sage, jasmine, rose, or German chamomile to ease mental fatigue and help you sleep better. Add 2 to 3 drops to a bowl of steaming water or add 5 to 6 drops to a bath.

CHINESE MEDICINE

There are several Chinese herbs that treat symptoms of depression. Aspiration is a combination of herbs that help relieve physical symptoms, constipation, loss of appetite and tightening in the chest. Gather Vitality is a combination of herbs that relieve sore limbs, fatigue or insomnia.

HERBAL REMEDIES

For mild depression, sip sage, ginseng, or powder bruised clover tea to relieve nausea and anxiety. (To make ginseng tea, boil 1 ounce fresh root with 1 cup of water for fifteen to twenty minutes. Drink up to two cups a day.) Spirulina eliminates toxins, rejuvenates, provides energy, regulates blood sugar. (Excess sugar in diet is linked to depression.) Drink tea made with the leaves and flowers of St. John's wort (no more than three cups a day), which acts as an antidepressant. Other teas you should try include ginger (for digestive problems), peppermint (for insomnia and anxiety), borage (for inflammation), and lemon balm and skullcap (for relaxation and reducing anxiety).

Ginkgo biloba leaves (in tea) improve blood flow to the brain. If you're taking Prozac or Zoloft, take St. John's wort 300 milligrams 3 times a day. Or try mixing two parts St. John's wort with one part oat, one part lavender, and one part mugwort. Take 5 milliliters three times a day for one month.

MIND-BODY

Follow Dr. Barnes's philosophy and get to know yourself (see sidebar page 241), your boundaries, and your limits. Establish a connection with your family. Depressed people tend to think negatively; try to focus on positive thoughts and memories. Depressed people want to be isolated, but the support of others can be a lifeline. Don't be afraid to reach out for help.

Exercise is a key to getting better. Even if you've never touched a barbell, start by walking outside or around your office building.

Depression is a signal you're not treating yourself right. It causes you to slow down and take notice, which can be a good thing. Get rid of that "got to do everything now" mentality. Charge ahead on some tasks; relax on others. Moderation is the key. Meditate, and repeat self-affirmations like "I am magnificent" or "I am wonderful" regularly; focus on finding and creating reasons to believe it.

Biofeedback is also helpful in treating depression—it teaches you how to stay in control of situations by regulating certain body functions, such as your heart rate, muscle tension, and temperature. Meditation, progressive muscle relaxation, yoga, and imagery help lift your mood, but also help you relax.

NUTRITION AND DIET

Make sure you're getting enough B vitamins (particularly if you're aged sixty to sixty-five, ask your doctor if you have B_{12} or folate deficiency), vitamin C, and folic acid. Try to eat regular meals at regular times even though you may not feel like eating. Vary your diet and limit your fat intake. Eat more vegetables, fruits, whole grains, cereals, beans, fish, poultry, and soy products, which contain tryptophan (which increases the production of serotonin, a hormone that releases chemicals in the brain that make us feel happy). Also, increase fiber and cut down on meat, sugar, caffeine, and junk food.

Prevention

Learn how to prioritize so you don't become overwhelmed. This will leave time to do the things you enjoy. Get adequate rest and exercise. Eat a healthy diet. If you have persistent bouts of depression or ever have suicidal thoughts, contact a qualified professional immediately.

 Testimonial

Denise R. Barnes, Ph.D., a clinical psychologist in private practice in Durham, North Carolina, preaches this holistic philosophy: Find balance in your life—spiritually, emotionally, physically, and mentally. "You must learn to connect with others, to become part of something that's bigger than you," says Dr. Barnes. The therapist also believes in patients' identifying obtainable, measurable goals not only to treat depression, but also as a life strategy. "Break down major goals into small steps—it makes it so much easier," she says. "I worked with a woman who was depressed and showed her how to do this. The more she broke her goals down, the more she was able to do, and slowly her depression eased."

Diabetes

Diabetes, or "sugar," as it's known to many African Americans, is a condition where the body produces little or no insulin (the hormone needed to transform carbohydrates into energy), causing sugar to accumulate in the blood, or the body produces plenty of insulin but excess body weight (or other factors) prevents its use. The types include insulin-dependent (type 1, which usually begins in childhood and requires regular intake of insulin) and noninsulin-dependent diabetes (type 2, which usually begins later in life and is more common). Someone with diabetes might experience these symptoms: frequent urination, thirst, hunger, blurred vision, yeast infections, impotence, vaginal infections, recurrent infections, fatigue, nausea or vomiting, or weight loss.

There are many long-term complications of diabetes such as blindness, circulatory problems, kidney and heart problems, as well as resistance to infections. Type 1 diabetes is believed to be caused by heredity and type 2 may be more prevalent in obese people and those over age forty. Gestational diabetes sometimes develops in pregnant women.

Statistics

For every six White Americans with diabetes, ten African Americans have the disease. Among African Americans in every age group more women than men have diabetes.

Treatments

ACUPUNCTURE

Acupuncture may relieve pain caused by the deterioration of the nervous system, strengthen the immune system, and keep the circulatory system in working order.

CHINESE MEDICINE

Ask an Oriental medical doctor about the following: lilyturg root, ginseng root, grassy privet, lotus seed, and Chinese yam.

HERBAL REMEDIES

Onion and garlic lower blood sugar and blood pressure and keep cholesterol levels down. Eat lots of cooked and raw garlic or take garlic capsules. Fenugreek seed and burdock (take as a powder) can also reduce blood sugar levels. Cayenne pepper cream may relieve pain associated with peripheral neuropathy (nerve degeneration common with diabetes). *Ginkgo biloba* (take as an extract) can increase blood flow and improve circulation in legs. Blueberry (take as fresh leaves in a decoction), may lower glucose levels and keep blood vessels strong.

MIND-BODY

Regular exercise is a key factor in managing your diabetes. It reduces the need for insulin injections, prevents the accumulation of cholesterol, and limits weight gain. It also increases tissue levels of chromium, which regulate blood glucose and cholesterol levels. **If you have type 1 diabetes, eat a bagel or high-energy snack before exercising to prevent hypoglycemia.** Aerobic exercise (swimming, aerobics, walking, bicycling) is beneficial if done for at least thirty minutes, three times a week. **If you have type 2 diabetes, avoid weightlifting or exertion activities that raise blood pressure and may aggravate eye problems.** You might try meditation, biofeedback, and other relaxation techniques to lower stress.

NUTRITION AND DIET

Many holistic practitioners attribute the high rate of diabetes (particularly among Blacks) to our diets, which include a lot of processed and refined foods. For noninsulin-dependent diabetes, eat a diet with high-fiber, whole-grain complex carbohydrates (50 to 60 percent); more fish, chicken, and soy products, and fewer red meats; lots of beans, peas, olive oil, root vegetables, cucumbers, garlic, soy beans, tofu, avocados, and brussels sprouts. Replace whole milk with nonfat milk; avoid all sugary foods, sweet fruits and juices; avoid alcohol and caffeine; take 2 tablespoons brewer's yeast per day. Also include vitamins B_6, B_{12}, C, manganese, zinc, and potassium in foods or supplements to treat deterioration of the nervous system, lower insulin needs for type 2 diabetics, strengthen the immune system, control blindness, metabolize glucose, increase tolerance for glucose, reduce the risk of heart problems, and maintain good cholesterol levels. Chromium, which is found in poultry, lean meats, brewer's yeast, whole grains, and eggs, as well as supplements, helps to regulate blood sugar levels and lowers insulin and cholesterol levels.

Prevention

Keep your weight in a healthy range. Exercise regularly, eat a nutritious diet. Don't smoke. Take good care of your teeth, gums, and feet. Complications from diabetes can be extremely serious, even life-threatening. It is critical to have regular checkups with your physician to monitor your condition.

Fibroid Tumors

For women, fibroid tumors can cause prolonged pain and discomfort. Fibroids, which are growths of noncancerous tissue, are found on the outside or inside wall of the uterus (womb). A woman with fibroids will experience these symptoms: painful intercourse, heavy or prolonged menstrual periods, anemia, constipation, fatigue, backache, pelvic pain, bloating, and frequent urination. Fibroids grow slowly and can change size and shape. They usually are seen in women in their late twenties to midforties. Many women have fibroid tumors without knowing it; the growths usually show no symptoms until they become very large or interfere with the workings of the uterus. Although their cause is unknown, fibroids have been linked to heredity, obesity, and hormonal imbalance, namely, too much estrogen. Fibroids occur most often in women who haven't had children or those who have taken birth control pills with high levels of estrogen.

Statistics

African American women are more than twice as likely as White women to develop fibroid tumors. They are also more likely than White women to be treated with a hysterectomy rather than hormone medication (which can shrink fibroids) or myomectomy (surgery that removes the tumor but keeps the uterus intact).

Treatments

ACUPUNCTURE/CHINESE MEDICINE

Try acupuncture and talk with an Oriental medical doctor about drinking a tea made of tao ren and hong hua. Also, the herb xiao liu pian (Tumor Reducing Tablet) has been shown to reduce the size of fibroids.

HERBAL REMEDIES

Naturopaths suggest some of the following treatments you can try: uterine tonics made of black cohosh and blue cohosh to help the general health and vitality of the uterus; cleavers (Galium aparine) often relieve health problems associated with benign growths; antispasmodics (black cohosh) lessen cramping; and lymphatics (cleavers, or Galium aparine) support drainage of fluid from uterus. To make a tea from cleavers, take it dried and drink 3 cups a day. As a tincture, take 2 to 4 milliliters three times a day. You also might try wild yam (take as a dried root, tincture, or capsule) for cramps; and chaste berry (to make a tea, pour 1 cup boiling water on 1 teaspoon berries). Infuse for ten to fifteen minutes. Drink raspberry leaf three times a day (use the dried leaf in a tea) or damiana (take as a tincture or capsule) to reduce fibroids.

HOMEOPATHY

Seek out a homeopath who might prescribe pulsatilla, belladonna, or sepia to relieve symptoms.

MASSAGE

Massage helps to release toxins in the muscles. It is also an excellent stress reliever. (Stress is considered a key contributor to fibroid tumor growth.)

MIND-BODY

To reduce the size of fibroids or sometimes eliminate them completely over time, make it a practice to lie or sit in a relaxed position in a quiet place. Focus your attention on the area of the fibroids and experience how you feel. Try to create an image of them, and focus. Allow that image to change. Try to form an image of something that could help them shrink. Visualize what your uterus looks like without fibroids.

Stress plays a major role in the development and recurrence of fibroids; it may upset your estrogen and progesterone balance. Practice stress-reduction techniques such as meditation and deep-breathing exercises: lie or sit in a comfortable position, and close your eyes and breathe deeply. Let your breathing become slow and relaxed. Focus only on your breathing. Notice the movement of your chest and abdomen, in and out. Say the word "rest" as you inhale. Say the word "relax" as you exhale. Draw out the pronunciation of each word so it lasts for the entire breath. Repeat these words several times. Repeat this exercise until you feel relaxed. Aerobic exercise for thirty minutes, at least three times a week, will keep your body in shape. Yoga and biofeedback therapy help you learn how to reduce the pain. Perhaps you might try affirmations (sit in a comfortable position, and tell your body that it is a well, fully functional system—use your own words, of course—and repeat three times). Or give these a try: progressive muscle relaxation and stretches to release muscle tension (especially in the abdominal area and lower back; these are good for menstrual cramps, too).

NUTRITION AND DIET

Cut back on red meat, chicken, and other dietary sources of estrogen. If you are overweight, have a sluggish metabolism, or have problems with mucus congestion, lay off the dairy, red meat, salt, and heavy foods (like turkey with dressing and all the fixins). If the liver, which breaks down estrogen, becomes sluggish or overworked, excess estrogen can build up. So go easy on your liver by avoiding fats, caffeine, and alcohol or any other drugs. A combination of herbs and amino acids can help the liver detoxify more efficiently (see a holistic practitioner for specific dosages). For good measure, take a multivitamin and mineral supplement. If you're bleeding heavily, make sure you haven't become anemic, which might mean you should add iron supplements, too. Castor oil packs to the abdomen may help your fibroids. (Soak a cloth with castor oil, apply to the abdomen and cover with plastic wrap and a towel. Apply a heating pad or hot water bottle on top of the pack for twenty to thirty minutes).

Bulk up on high-fiber foods (vegetables, fruits, whole grains) to help reduce estrogen production and bring your hormones back in balance. Get more vitamin C and the bioflavonoids found in citrus fruits, leafy vegetables, and red onions. Get more vitamin E from wheat germ, vegetable oils, seeds, and nuts. Get more vitamin A from liver, kidney, and low-fat milk. Also, drink plenty of water.

Ayurvedic medicine contends that if you are bleeding heavily, you probably have a fire (pitta) imbalance. Avoid hot, spicy, acidic, and sour food, and avoid hot tubs. Try a macrobiotic diet: lots of whole grains, beans, vegetables, and occasional fruits.

Prevention

Eliminate meat (yes, those juicy T-bone steaks) and dairy products from your diet. These contain hormones such as estrogen that are used to stimulate growth in farm animals, and may contribute to fibroids. Replace them with beans, nuts, and leafy green vegetables. Also, cut back on coffee, tea, chocolate, cola, salt, alcohol, fried foods, and foods high in sugar.

Chill. Release anger and anxiety with deep-breathing exercises or meditation. And get some exercise while you're at it!

See your physician for regular pelvic examinations once a year. The high rate of fibroids among Black women may be due to the fact that they wait too long to see their gynecologist or don't get regular checkups.

 Testimonial

Beverly Lomax, 61, of Philadelphia, Pennsylvania, discovered she had fibroid tumors after a routine Pap smear examination. "They found a large fibroid about the size of a four-month-old baby," Lomax recalls. She began experiencing severe bleeding, and her physician recommended a hysterectomy, which she decided against. While she was taking medication to stop the bleeding and restore her hormones, Lomax began researching alternative healing. She followed a semi-macrobiotic diet that included beans, brown rice, fruit, foods high in iron, and very little meat or chicken. "I also meditated, prayed, and practiced visualization three times a day. I had shiatsu massages once a week to loosen the toxins in my body," she recalls. "I saw small changes in a few months; after a year when I went back to my gynecologist, the fibroids had gone down a good bit. And on my next visit about two years later, they were nearly gone."

Glaucoma

A disease that steals your sight before you realize what has happened is another condition that's all too familiar to African Americans. Glaucoma is the build up of fluid resulting in pressure inside the eye, which can lead to eventual damage to the optic nerve, causing a slow, painless loss of your peripheral (side) vision. If untreated, glaucoma can progress into total blindness. Often, no symptoms appear until late stages, when symptoms include eyes aching, tearing, blurred vision, headaches, redness, dilated pupils, throbbing pain in and above the eye, gradual loss of peripheral vision, and the perception of rainbow rings around lights. There are several types of glaucoma, including chronic, or open-angle glaucoma (causes no symptoms in early stages); acute, or closed-angle glaucoma (rapid rise in painful eye pressure); and congenital, which is extremely rare and occurs only in newborns.

Chronic glaucoma, the most common form, develops as a person ages. It appears that heredity is the cause of acute glaucoma, which occurs when the iris of the eye blocks normal drainage channels and fluid pressure builds up. Congenital glaucoma is caused by a defect in the drainage angle present before birth. You may be at risk for glaucoma if you use some antidepressants or steroids at length, which build pressure in the eye. Also, corticosteroid eye drops destroy collagen, a protein that keeps eye tissue healthy. If you have allergies, are over age forty, nearsighted, are under a lot of stress, or have hypertension (affects your blood vessels) or diabetes you may be prone to glaucoma, too. In fact, diabetes, which affects the circulatory system, triples your risk of developing glaucoma.

Statistics
Glaucoma is the leading cause of blindness in African Americans, who are ten times more likely to develop glaucoma blindness than Whites. It also occurs earlier in Blacks than in Whites. More than 2 million Black Americans have glaucoma. Many factors, including heredity or environmental factors, and the disproportionate presence of hypertension and diabetes in the Black community explain its prevalence among us.

Treatments

ACUPUNCTURE

Acupuncture may help to relieve tension and pressure that builds up in the eye. Consult a trained acupuncturist, who will target points in the areas of the gallbladder, liver, and kidney meridians.

AYURVEDIC MEDICINE

Glaucoma is a disorder of the kapha dosha, so a practitioner is likely to prescribe punarnava to reduce pressure or tell you to avoid white sugar, coffee, and dairy products. You could also prepare a tea made from the herb (steep 1 teaspoon of herb in 1 cup of hot water for two minutes. Strain until herb disappears from water, and drink two to three times a day). Be sure to talk to your ophthalmologist before seeing an Ayurvedic medicine practitioner.

HERBAL REMEDIES

Marijuana has been proven to reduce pressure associated with glaucoma. While it is an illegal substance, it can be legally prescribed by a physician for glaucoma patients. Try taking 2 to 4 ounces of bilberry berries three times a day to maintain collagen levels.

MIND-BODY

Try these eye exercises for eyestrain: Sit in a comfortable position, breathe deeply, and cover your eyes with the palms of your hands. Or take several deep breaths and then roll your head around in a circular motion and stretch your neck and shoulders, then move your head side to side, up and down, repeating two or three times. Also try applying a hot cloth to your eyes for three minutes, then apply a cold cloth and alternate two to three times.

NUTRITION AND DIET

Eating a healthy diet can help your condition. Take vitamin C (as supplements—up to 3,000 milligrams a day—and found in cauliflower, broccoli, turnip greens, strawberries, and citrus fruits) or omega-3 fatty acids to reduce pressure and restore collagen levels to normal. Increase your intake of bioflavonoids (which strengthen capillaries and other tissues of the eye), which are found in citrus fruits, leafy vegetables, red onions, beets, blue or red berries; and vitamin A, which is found in liver, egg yolk, butter, cheese, dairy products, or cod liver oil. Take zinc, chromium and vitamin B_1, which those with glaucoma often lack. Also, reduce your intake of alcohol and caffeine (interferes with circulation to the eye).

REFLEXOLOGY

Eliminating toxins, and breaking down and eliminating pressure inside the eyeball can help. Consult a reflexologist who is likely to focus on the eye, neck, kidney, throat and diaphragm reflexes on your feet. Or try this yourself: Massage at the base of the second and third toes on your left foot, just below where they join your sole.

Prevention

Get a comprehensive eye examination every other year or every year if you are at risk. Eat healthily, drink bottled water, and lay off the tobacco smoke. Also, actively work to avoid hypertension and diabetes, or if you have either condition or both, keep it under control.

Gynecological/Menstrual Problems

The reproductive system of a woman is extremely complex. And as with any system, is prone to "breakdowns" or "malfunctions" from time to time.

Amenorrhea is a condition characterized by irregular or absent periods caused by dieting, eating disorders, stress, excessive exercising, birth control pills, or depression.

Dysmenorrhea is a condition characterized by stomach cramps, bloating, and tender breasts associated with menstruation. It is common in young women just starting their periods and is triggered by changes in the menstrual cycle that cause the uterus to contract.

Endometriosis is a condition characterized by back or abdominal pain and heavy menstrual bleeding. It is caused by fragments of uterine lining that shed during menstruation and settle on or near reproductive organs.

Menorrhagia is a condition characterized by periods lasting more than five days with excessive bleeding. It can be caused by fibroids, or the use of an intrauterine device (IUD).

Pelvic inflammatory disease is an infection of the female reproductive organs sometimes resulting from sexually transmitted diseases, abortion, or miscarriage. The symptoms include pelvic pain, fever, or foul-smelling discharge.

Premenstrual syndrome (PMS) is a condition characterized by emotional and/or physical discomfort before or during the first day or two of your period. Symptoms include depression, sadness, irritability, anger, fatigue, bloating, breast tenderness, weight gain, food cravings, insomnia, head, back, or stomach pain.

Statistics

Nine out of ten women, including Black women, experience some discomfort during their periods, including cramps, headache, nausea, bloating, and/or breast tenderness. About one in ten experience severe or incapacitating cramps. Endometriosis occurs in 7 to 15 percent of women and is more common in Whites than Blacks.

Treatments

ACUPUNCTURE/CHINESE MEDICINE

Chinese medicine asserts that there are two organs that regulate menstruation, the Liver and Spleen. When there is disharmony in the Liver, you feel emotional swings associated with PMS. When there's disruption in the Spleen, you experience distention of abdomen and breasts, and insomnia. Excessive dairy products, greasy or fried foods, emotional strain, and overwork can all lead to PMS. Acupuncture and herbs (Xiao Yao Wan that contains Dang Gui) relieve PMS, usually after a minimum of three menstrual periods. Meditation, Tai Chi, or Qi Gong (breathing exercises to amplify and invigorate *chi* energy) help relieve the root of the problem.

Dysmenorrhea is said to come from a lack of blood in the body or stagnant *chi* or blood, which affects emotions. Acupuncture treatment involves freeing up stagnant *chi* and blood, and nourishing and increasing the amount of blood circulating to remove pain and ease emotions.

AROMATHERAPY
For cramps, add 3 drops each of essential oil of chamomile and sweet marjoram to 2 teaspoons carrier oil or lotion. Massage into skin or add to warm bath.

CHIROPRACTIC
Adjustment reduces discomfort in lower back, releases endorphins, and relieves pressure on nerves. Endorphins are proteins in the brain that release chemicals that make us feel calm and relaxed.

FOLK REMEDIES
For cramps, drink hot herbal teas (sage, nutmeg, or ginger work well), apply a hot water bottle to your abdomen, or soak in a warm bath. Warm ginger ale is said to help thin out blood clots. To avoid headaches and fatigue associated with menstruation, eat bananas a week before your period and sweet potatoes during the week after it.

HERBAL REMEDIES
There are many herbal remedies to address gynecological problems. Some specific ones you can try are red raspberry, blue cohosh,

and dong quai for cramps and bloating. Or you can try this: Blend clary sage (a natural source of estrogen), patchouli, cinnamon stick (a uterine stimulant), vitamin E, myrrh (cleanses the reproductive tract), and carrier oil with coconut oil (contact a naturopath for the specific recipe). Blend together in a glass (not plastic) container. Roll between your palms; don't shake. Use this as a lotion for the abdominal area to soothe the symptoms of PMS or endometriosis.

Also good for PMS: vitamin B_6; vitamin E (for breast tenderness); magnesium (for breast tenderness, tension, and weight gain); and primrose oil during menstruation (for breast tenderness, depression, and irritability).

Cramp bark relaxes muscular tension and spasms. Try this: Add 2 teaspoons dried bark to 1 cup water. Simmer fifteen minutes. Drink this hot three times a day. You might want to also try this recipe:

Add 1 cup hot water to 1 teaspoon grated fresh ginger root; steep for ten minutes and drink as needed to relieve cramps.

For heavy periods, try American cranesbill or periwinkle for excessive blood loss: pour 1 cup boiling water on 1 teaspoon of either herb. Steep for fifteen minutes and drink three times a day.

For pelvic inflammatory disease, eat raw garlic or take three garlic capsules three times a day.

Also, raspberry leaf, black currant, yarrow and chamomile teas may be soothing for dysmenorrhea.

HOMEOPATHY

Here is a sampling of some homeopathic treatments for menstrual problems:

If you are experiencing cramps that seem to be relieved only when you are bending over or when you apply pressure, you should consider Colocynthis 6C (Bitter Cucumber). Not only is it indicated for cramps and twitching, but it is suitable in situations in women experiencing constrictions and contractions. Chamomilla

6C (Chamomile) is excellent if your cramps seem like labor pains and reach an unbearable level.

Women whose menstrual cramps make the individual miserable should turn to Sepia 6C (Cuttlefish), one of the most important uterine remedies.

For heavy menstrual flow, you can select from:

• Cina 6C (Worm-Seed)—dark clotty flow with spasms

• Belladonna 6C (Nightshade)—bright red profuse flow

• Ipecac 6C (Ipecac-Root)—heavy flow with nausea

For PMS use either Sepia 6C (Cuttlefish); Pulsatilla 6C (Wind Flower); Nux Vomica 6C (Poison-Nut).

MASSAGE

For cramps, massage your lower abdomen, lower back, and legs. Start with the uterus to relieve spasms and stimulate blood flow. Lie on the floor with your knees bent. Put your right arm on the lower right side of your abdomen and put your left hand on top of your right arm. Press with all of your fingers, making small circular motions. Move your hands up the right side of your abdomen to your waist, across and under your ribs and down again, across your lower abdomen above your pubic hair. Have a friend massage your legs and back using large, upward stroking movements.

MIND-BODY

For endometriosis, visualizing at least twice a day can be beneficial. Sit or lie quietly and start breathing deeply, filling out your stomach. Relax each part of your body part by part, head to toe. When relaxed, visualize yourself in pleasant surroundings, then envision the weak endometriosis cells being attacked by the strong white blood cells. Imagine scar tissue disintegrating; visualize healthy internal organs.

Regular moderate exercise prevents fluid retention, relaxes your muscles, improves blood flow for PMS symptoms, and also stimulates endorphins, which are proteins in the brain that release chemicals which make us feel calm and relaxed. For dysmenorrhea, you might find that yoga, aerobic exercise, and stretching relieve cramps.

NUTRITION AND DIET

For PMS, take vitamin B_6, and/or a daily B-complex tablet; vitamin C; vitamin E; vitamin A; calcium; magnesium; chromium; zinc; and DL-phenylalanine to relieve symptoms. Try to eat a high carbohydrate diet and decrease salt, sugar, fat, processed foods, caffeine, and alcohol.

For endometriosis, take vitamin B_6, with 25 to 50 milligrams vitamin B complex per day; vitamin E; a multivitamin and mineral supplement with calcium and magnesium (to reduce the pain of cramps), and vitamin E (keeps scar tissue soft). You'll need to decrease dairy, sweets, caffeine, salt, and animal fats; and bulk up on fiber.

An effective way to relieve cramps is by eating sardines, salmon, mackerel, or by taking fish oil supplements, which help combat the production of muscle-cramping prostaglandins; or taking vitamin B_6, and vitamin B complex.

For heavy periods, take more iron and zinc (found in red meat, poultry, fish, and green, leafy vegetables, or 50 milligrams a day supplements). Try to eat or drink citrus fruits and juices with meals for better iron absorption. Take vitamin B_6 and B complex. Get vitamin A through supplements or food (liver, kidney, egg yolk, butter, whole milk, cod liver oil). Take bioflavonoids (found in red onions, citrus fruits, and leafy vegetables) and vitamin C.

For amenorrhea, eat foods rich in vitamin B_6 (found in lean meat, wheat germ, and brewer's yeast) or take supplements of vitamin B_6 with one 25-milligram vitamin B complex; and eat plenty of foods rich in zinc.

For pelvic inflammatory disease, eat lots of vitamin C, vitamin A, and vitamin D from foods or supplements, whole-grain cereals, lean meats, fish, and green, leafy vegetables. Eat live yogurt cultures with *Lactobacillus acidophilus* to prevent thrush if you're taking antibiotics.

Prevention

For amenorrhea, try to maintain a healthy amount of body fat for your age and height. This means maintaining a reasonable weight and not overdoing the aerobic exercise. For endometriosis, use sanitary napkins instead of tampons, which may block menstrual flow. For PMS, avoid caffeine, sweets, tea, soft drinks, chocolate, and alcohol. You need to eat nutritiously to maintain your blood sugar level. Try to exercise, reduce your stress levels, and get extra sleep one week before your period. You also need to drink plenty of fluids, eat plenty of fruit and hold off on the salt shaker.

Headaches

Many of us reach for the aspirin or Tylenol bottle when we feel that familiar throbbing or pounding in our heads and need relief. Here we offer some natural remedies to cure headaches. Tension headaches, which are the most common form of headache, are characterized by pain and tightness around the head. They are caused by tightened muscles of the scalp, neck, face, or shoulders. Symptoms include dull pain, and tightness around the scalp and neck.

Migraines are severe headaches often accompanied by nausea and vomiting, and preceded by depression and irritability. Symptoms include nausea, vomiting, lightheadedness, reduced field of vision, sensation of flashing lights, and pain on one side of the head.

Cluster headaches are characterized by pain around or behind the eye with several attacks occurring one after the other for days, weeks, or months, then disappearing completely for one year or more. Symptoms include sudden pain around or behind the eye, nasal congestion, and a flushed face.

Sinus headaches are characterized by inflammation or infection of membranes lining the sinus cavities caused by hay fever, allergies, cold, or the flu. Symptoms include nasal congestion, eye pain, and pressure behind the face.

Causes vary depending on the type of headache, but generally include fatigue, depression, hunger, dehydration, caffeine withdrawal, food additives (especially MSG), allergies, sinusitis, tension and strain in neck, facial and head muscles from poor posture or stress, low blood sugar, change in daily routine, weather changes, bright light, loud sounds, or prolonged staring at a computer or television.

Statistics

Forty-five million Americans regularly have severe headaches requiring medical attention each year, according to the National Headache Foundation.

Treatments

ACUPRESSURE

Here's something you can do to relieve pain from sinus headaches: Place both index fingers at the bottom of your cheekbones with your fingertips under your eyes. Press firmly for one minute and repeat three times. Or to reduce stress in your neck causing a tension headache, place the tips of your middle fingers in the hollow area at the base of your skull about two inches apart, on both sides of your spine and press firmly for one minute.

ACUPUNCTURE/CHINESE MEDICINE

According to Chinese medicine, causes for headaches range from phlegm, blood stasis, deficiency of *chi* and blood, to Liver Yang Rising or invasion of pathogenic (causing disease) wind into the meridians and collaterals. Depending on the cause, acupuncture can bring relief by resolving the phlegm, moving the blood, or pacifying the liver.

AROMATHERAPY

For tension headaches, put one to two drops of essential oil of lavender onto your fingertips and massage in a circular motion across your temples, behind your ears, around eyes, and across the back of your neck for relief. Use the same technique, but with eucalyptus for a sinus headache. Also, applying lavender, rosemary, and peppermint in a compress to your head, poured into your bath, or inhaled are useful for any type of headache.

CHIROPRACTIC

Tension headaches can be caused by poor posture that puts unnecessary strain on your muscles. A chiropractor can manipulate or realign the spine or cervix. Sometimes a chiropractor will look for possible links to nitrates (found in bacon, some cheeses, bologna, onions, and chocolate), which cause an allergic reaction in some people.

HERBAL REMEDIES

According to some herbalists, the following are remedies for headaches you can make: Sip hot ginger tea to relax blood vessels in your head: Stir 500 to 600 mg powdered or 1 teaspoon grated fresh ginger into 6 ounces of boiling water and cool before drinking. (Ginger activates the natural opiates in the brain that relieve pain while reducing chemicals that cause inflammation.) Other good teas to try include chamomile, lemon balm, rose hips, and linden (from the lime tree—improves blood circulation in migraines and vascular headaches).

To reduce tension, drink valerian tea: pour 1 cup boiling water onto 2 teaspoons of root. Steep for fifteen minutes and drink before bedtime. Also, cool any of these teas, pour onto a clean cloth, and use as a compress on your forehead.

Try this compress to soothe throbbing temples: add essential oil of peppermint, eucalyptus and lavender to cold or warm water. Soak a cloth with the mixture; wring it well. Put the cloth over your forehead and eyes while lying down for ten minutes and repeat if needed.

Sinus headaches can be relieved with goldenseal, taken as a tincture, tea or powder three times a day.

Tincture of feverfew leaves and *Ginkgo biloba* leaves reduce vascular headaches, including migraines. Drinking tea or taking a tincture made from hawthorn, skullcap, and cramp bark three times a day also helps ease migraines caused by stress.

HOMEOPATHY

One of the finest remedies for headaches that come on suddenly and intensely is Belladonna 6C (Nightshade). Kali Bichronmicum 6C (Bichromate of Potash) is especially indicated for aching headaches that blur the vision.

MASSAGE

To relieve tension in your scalp, neck, and facial muscles, use your fingertips, and massage your scalp, pretending you're washing your hair.

MIND-BODY

You should exercise regularly to prevent tension in your neck and shoulder muscles, dilate blood vessels, which increases blood flow and prevents migraines from occurring, and releases endorphins, hormones in the brain that release chemicals stimulating a sense of well-being. Also try walking, swimming, or jogging. Meditation, biofeedback, and progressive relaxation can do wonders for reducing stress, which is linked to tension headaches.

NUTRITION AND DIET

Avoid foods that contain amines (chemicals that dilate blood vessels) such as cabbage, eggplant, bananas, potatoes, tomatoes, canned fish, wine, beer, and cured meat. Avoid foods that can trigger an allergic reaction such as cheddar or Brie cheese, onions, soy, wheat, yeast, grapes, oranges, peanuts, rice, fish, eggs, milk, corn, sugar, apples, and beef. You should also avoid coffee, black tea, alcohol, MSG, and Aspartame (artificial sweetener). Take omega-3 fatty acids niacin, and magnesium.

Check to see if you have food sensitivities to wheat, corn, or dairy. Avoid refined flour and simple sugar. Make sure you're not hypoglycemic. Also, eat small meals during the day and drink adequate amounts of water (eight glasses a day).

Prevention

Avoid MSG and excessive caffeine and alcohol, and eat nutritious meals at regular times to avoid low blood sugar. Taper off caffeine gradually if you're trying to cut back, catch plenty of zzz's, avoid stress if you can, exercise, and get outside. If you think the headache stems from something you ate or did, keep a daily food/activity diary and note possible food/activity triggers. If you're a woman, determine if migraines are connected to hormonal changes associated with your menstrual cycle.

There are times when a headache can be a symptom of a more serious problem. Here are some warning signs of a dangerous headache: If your headache persists over several days, is associated with a fall or other trauma, occurs daily, is sudden and excruciating, is accompanied by fever and stiff neck, or is associated with difficulty hearing, seeing, speaking or moving an arm or leg—call your doctor.

Heart Disorders

Fred Sanford of the popular television show *Sanford & Son* was always clutching his chest, pretending he was having a heart attack. But heart attacks and heart problems are no joke. Take note of these remedies to possibly prevent you from having a heart attack. Angina occurs when the heart is deprived of the necessary amount of oxygen due to blocked or narrowed coronary arteries. It is sometimes confused with indigestion. Angina can be brought on by chest pain during overexertion, stress or anxiety. It is often a warning sign of coronary heart disease. Symptoms include pain in the center of the chest, which can spread to the upper jaw, throat, back, or left arm. **Note:** Symptoms of heart disease can indicate a medical emergency. Consult a physician immediately if you experience chest pain or discomfort.

Atherosclerosis is the hardening and narrowing of arteries, caused by fatty cholesterol-rich deposits that accumulate on the inner lining of blood vessels. There usually are no symptoms until a major health crisis occurs such as a stroke, kidney failure, angina, or a heart attack.

Coronary heart disease is the narrowing or blocking of the arteries supplying the heart muscle. It causes angina and may lead to a heart attack.

Congestive heart failure is the gradual loss of the heart's ability to pump blood efficiently. In this condition, fluid accumulates in the veins that carry blood from the lungs, causing the lungs and legs to become swollen and congested. Symptoms include breathlessness, fatigue, chest pain, loss of appetite, mental confusion, and frequent urination.

Statistics

In 1991, deaths from cardiovascular disease were 47 percent higher for African American men compared to White men, and 69 percent higher in African American women compared to White women.

Treatments

AROMATHERAPY
Aromatherapy can help you unwind—add four to five drops of lavender oil to a bath or steam inhalation (avoid this if you have asthma), or sprinkle two drops on a tissue and inhale.

CHINESE MEDICINE
Angina is considered a stagnation of the blood and energy in the heart. Herbal medicines such as cinnamon twigs, safflower, red sage root, or macrosten onion bulb may help. Consult an Oriental medical doctor for specific remedies.

HERBAL REMEDIES
Hot red peppers (found in chili or the herb capsicum) may help prevent blood clots. Onions and garlic also can be beneficial to you by helping to reduce blood clotting. Fresh ginger helps reduce the stickiness of blood platelets and thus reduces clotting. An infusion of hawthorn berries is a good tonic: Pour 1 cup of water on 2 teaspoons hawthorn berries and steep for twenty minutes and drink three times a day (warm or cold).

MIND-BODY
Exercise vigorously for a minimum of twenty to thirty minutes, three times a week to keep your heart pumping stronger and longer and to generate a healthy balance of HDL (good cholesterol) to LDL (bad cholesterol). Yoga and meditation greatly help reduce stress and induce relaxation. Biofeedback can also help you learn to chill out.

NUTRITION AND DIET

Enjoy at least five half-cup servings of fruits and vegetables (major sources of beta-carotene) daily. Vitamin C is believed to stop artery-clogging plaque in smokers and help heart attack victims, so take note if you fall in these categories. Eat lots of whole-grain cereals, oily fish (sardines, salmon, or herring), cooked dried beans and peas, and moderate amounts of poultry, nonfat milk and nonfat or low-fat cheeses that help keep your heart healthy and functioning properly. Adequate amounts of magnesium and vitamin E are also important for proper heart functioning. The coenzyme Q10 (taken as a supplement) prevents the accumulation of fatty acids within the heart muscle. The amino acid carnitine (taken as a supplement) improves the burning of fatty acids, thus improving the heart muscle's stress tolerance. It also helps lower your total cholesterol and triglyceride levels and prevents irregular heartbeat. Eat plenty of beta-carotene (found in carrots, squash, and sweet potatoes), a powerful antioxidant that reduces symptoms as well as the incidence of stroke and heart attacks.

Prevention

If you are overweight, try to lose those extra pounds—they put unneeded strain on the heart and raise blood cholesterol levels. Avoid fatty, red meat, whole-milk dairy products, sweets, fried foods, and salt, which clog arteries. Eat fewer eggs and cook with olive or canola oil instead of cholesterol-laden butter or lard. Stop smoking—it constricts blood vessels. Exercising is important to tone your heart and blood vessels and keep weight down. And surrender your stress—you'll feel less tense and anxious about things.

 Testimonial

Doris Jones, forty-six, of Oxon Hill, Maryland, knew she had to make some changes in her life after surviving a heart

attack in 1994. Jones had been a vegetarian for several years and was seeing a holistic practitioner, but still experienced circulation problems in her legs and feet. At her husband's suggestion, she sought out a reflexologist who helped her recover her strength. Today, she attributes her health to a holistic approach that combines a sound diet with herbs. "I take herbs and herbal teas for the heart, such as hawthorn berries, garlic, capsicum and *Ginkgo biloba*," Jones says. "I feel healthy and have a lot of energy when I eat vegetarian."

Hemorrhoids

One very painful, but common condition—hemorrhoids—can be relieved in a variety of ways. Hemorrhoids occur when varicose veins of the anus and lower rectum have become swollen and stretched. They are found either outside or inside the rectum. Symptoms include anal pain, burning, itching and bleeding, pain during bowel movements, painful swelling or a lump near the anus, or an anal mucus discharge. They tend to be hereditary. Hemorrhoids can be aggravated by straining during a bowel movement or hard stools that make the veins drain poorly and swell permanently. These swollen veins either rupture and bleed or press on surrounding nerves, producing the symptoms.

Hemorrhoids are caused by many things. Overweight people tend to get more hemorrhoids because the extra girth puts added pressure on the anal veins. (Not exercising and eating low-fiber foods hurts, too.) Other common causes include abusing laxatives, prolonged sitting or standing, straining from constipation or diarrhea, coughing, sneezing, resisting the urge to defecate (increases pressure in the bowel area), and pregnancy (because the expanding uterus puts added pressure on the anal veins).

Statistics

Approximately three of every four Blacks and Whites alike have hemorrhoids. Hemorrhoids occur in people mostly between the ages of twenty and fifty.

Treatments

AROMATHERAPY

For soothing relief, add to a warm bath four drops of peppermint and cypress essential oils, and 2 tablespoons bicarbonate of soda and sit and soak for thirty minutes to an hour.

HERBAL REMEDIES

Dab cotton balls or pads in witch hazel and apply to inflamed areas to cool things down. Herbal creams made from calendula, oil from St. John's wort, and butcher's broom ointment or suppositories are also helpful if you are in pain. For external hemorrhoids, apply pilewort ointment (simmer 2 teaspoons fresh or dried pilewort in 7 ounces petroleum jelly for ten minutes and cool) twice a day, or take as a tea.

HOMEOPATHY

Hemorrhoids present different symptoms in different people. The best-proven homeopathic remedies are:

- Ratanhia 6C (Krameria)—feeling like you are passing broken pieces of glass

- Hamamelis 6C (witch hazel)—sore and raw feeling in rectum

- Sepia 6C (Cuttlefish)—feeling of a ball in rectum

- Sulphur 6C (Sulphur)—itching, burning, with hard stools

MASSAGE

To relieve constipation, in the morning before eating, oil your hands lightly (preferably with olive oil). Lie down and place one hand on top of the other on your lower stomach. With your fingers flat against your skin, press down about 1 inch into your abdomen at the left corner. Make small, slow circles. Move your hands up (toward your head) slightly and repeat. Continue up your left side, across and above your navel, and down your right side. Repeat with large, slow sweeping strokes. Then go in the reverse direction, first with small circles, then with large strokes. Repeat two to three times.

MIND-BODY

It's important to take a brisk walk or a dance or exercise class to keep your digestive system functioning properly. You may also benefit from yoga, which decreases blood flow around hemorrhoids, reducing bleeding, pain, and inflammation.

NUTRITION AND DIET

To keep stools soft and bulky and to avoid excess strain on hemorrhoids, eat a fiber-rich diet including fresh fruits (apples, oranges, prunes, raisins); vegetables (cabbage, carrots, brussel sprouts, dark, leafy lettuce, corn); bran, whole-grain breads, oatmeal, beans (soy, kidney, lentils, lima), and brown rice. Add fiber to your diet gradually over several weeks to prevent gas, cramping, and diarrhea. Drink at least eight, 8-ounce glasses of water a day to help soften stools and maintain digestive flow. Avoid coffee, strong spices, beer, and cola—they're all irritants.

Prevention

Get more roughage (fiber) in your diet! Fiber prevents constipation and keeps you regular. Find a vigorous exercise you like and "just do it." Keep your weight down. Take frequent breaks from standing or sitting. Don't strain when you sit on the toilet and try not to stay there all day. Check with your doctor to rule out more serious conditions (such as colorectal cancer or dermatitis) that can also cause constipation.

Hyperactivity

You've probably met this child in your son or daughter's play group or maybe in your own family: the child who can't sit still, moving from room to room with lightning speed, or who has the attention span of about two seconds. Hyperactivity is a disorder of infants and children who are unusually overactive and restless. Hyperactive babies often cry nonstop, have eczema, and eat poorly. In school, these children are disruptive, unable to keep still, and fearful. They also have short attention spans, poor coordination, and tend to throw things. Young children with attention-deficit/ hyperactivity disorder (ADHD) are typically overactive, unable to pay attention, impulsive, and accident-prone. Older children or teenagers with the disorder may do poorly in school despite normal or above-normal intelligence. Hyperactivity is caused by heredity, allergies caused by excess sugar and milk, environmental factors, a poor diet, or lack of exercise. For children with ADHD, some doctors recommend stimulant drugs like Dexedrine, Ritalin and Cylert to activate the part of the brain that suppresses excess activity. However, these drugs also suppress appetite, slowing growth temporarily. Side effects of these drugs include nausea, abdominal pain, and weight loss. Ritalin is controversial because it is prescribed so frequently, particularly to African American children. Psychotherapy and assessment for special education may help you decide the best treatment for your child.

Statistics

As many as one in every twenty children have ADHD. Boys outnumber girls by three to one. African American males are disproportionately diagnosed with attention deficit disorder (ADD, which has similar symptoms to ADHD: difficulty concentrating, following directions, remembering events, tasks, or time), which also sends many of our boys to special education classes, sometimes inappropriately.

Treatments

AROMATHERAPY

To calm your child, put dried lavender or chamomile in a pillow to relieve nervousness and have him sleep on it or add to his bath for a relaxing experience.

HERBAL REMEDIES

Hyperactive children often lack essential fatty acids. These can be replenished by supplementing with evening primrose oil (read the label for a child's dosage). Rubbing the oil into the skin (1 ml oil twice a day) can help, too. You might also find these helpful: Catnip (take as an extract or infusion for irritability); cowslip (for nervous tension, take as an extract or tablet); chamomile (take for irritability as a tea or tincture); passion flower (take for irritability as an extract, tincture or tablet); valerian (take for excitability as an infusion, tincture or extract); and wild lettuce (take for excitability as an extract).

HOMEOPATHY

Homeopathy helps children with ADHD. Stimulant drugs can neutralize homeopathic remedies, so it's important to identify the symptoms in your child before medication and start with repeated low potencies. Controlling your child's diet and other environmental factors increases the effectiveness of therapy.

NUTRITION AND DIET

There's a clear link between hyperactivity and certain foods and food additives. Thus, eliminating these foods and medications from your child's diet may improve his or her condition: fast food, processed foods, snack foods (potato chips, pretzels, etc.), all foods and drinks with synthetic coloring, flavoring, and additives (the food coloring tartrazine [Yellow #5] is especially bad); all aspirin products and artificially flavored vitamin pills and children's medications; foods and drinks with sugar; any food your child is allergic to (common offenders: milk, corn, wheat, eggs); and in some instances, tap water (it can contain ingredients that cause hyperactivity, so use spring water instead). If your child is on Ritalin, Dexedrine, or other medications, make sure he or she gets plenty of fresh fruits and vegetables to round out his diet. Also, provide only low-fat dairy products, whole-grain breads and cereals, lean meats, or dried beans and peas. To completely ensure he's getting all the nutrients he needs, give him a multivitamin. Make sure your child gets vitamin B complex with vitamin B_3 added, vitamin C, and zinc, too—it helps hyperactivity. Read the label for a child's dosage.

Prevention

Although it's difficult to pinpoint a cause for ADHD, prevention can start as early as your pregnancy: get good prenatal care, stay away from alcohol, cigarettes and other harmful chemicals. Also, make sure your child receives good general health care.

Hypertension

Of all vascular disorders (blood vessels), high blood pressure, or hypertension, is the most common. Hypertension occurs when blood presses with excess force against the walls of the blood vessels. High blood pressure may damage the arteries and, in turn, the heart, kidneys, or brain, causing heart attack, kidney failure, stroke, or eye damage. Your blood pressure is considered high if it reads 140/90 or higher for people ages eighteen to sixty-four; and 160/90 or higher for people ages sixty-five and older. The first number represents the systolic pressure (when your heart squeezes); the second, the diastolic pressure (between beats when the heart rests). High blood pressure is called the "silent killer," because this condition usually causes no symptoms. Factors contributing to hypertension include stress, heredity, high-salt diets, oral contraceptives and pregnancy (because a mother's blood volume triples, placing additional strain on the heart).

Statistics

More than one out of three (38 percent) Black Americans have hypertension. Black males under age forty-five are ten times more likely than White males to die from hypertension-related illness. Overall, about 27 percent of women suffer from hypertension. Among postmenopausal Black women, the rate is close to 80 percent.

Treatments

ACUPRESSURE

These may help improve circulation and reduce high blood pressure if you try them. Find the point along your biceps tendon where your elbow creases, which is in line with your ring finger, and press firmly with your thumb for one minute, repeating on your other arm. Or press the point that's four finger-widths up from your inner anklebone, near the edge of your shinbone, with your thumb for one minute, and repeat on your other leg. **Do not do if pregnant.**

AROMATHERAPY

Lavender aids relaxation. Add a few drops to your bath.

CHINESE MEDICINE

If you were to seek out an Oriental medicine doctor, he or she would prescribe remedies containing the following: chrysanthemum flower, ginseng, peony root, and astragalus to help lower blood pressure.

FOLK REMEDY

To help reduce your blood pressure, chop one garlic clove into small pieces. Place it on a spoon and take with a glass of water. Repeat two to three times a day.

HERBAL REMEDIES

To help reduce high blood pressure, dilate blood vessels, and moderate heart rate, take hawthorn as a tea (steep dried flowers and berries of the herb in hot water for ten to fifteen minutes).

MASSAGE

Regular massage helps relieve stress and tension and lower blood pressure. You can teach yourself or your mate and practice, practice, practice.

MIND-BODY

Prayer, meditation, yoga, relaxation tapes, and biofeedback (teaches you to control body responses such as temperature or heart rate so you can relax) can help reduce or eliminate stress. First, figure out what's pushing your buttons. If you're working too much, cut back if you can. Get more sleep. Or try this relaxation exercise: Find a quiet place and lie on your back. Close your eyes, allow your breathing to slow, and begin to notice how your body feels. Try to relax every body part beginning with your face, working down to your toes. This should take about ten minutes. If all else fails, do something you enjoy—that's relaxing!

NUTRITION AND DIET

Eat at least three to four servings a day of potassium-rich foods, to lower your blood pressure. These include low-fat dairy products, fish, and virtually all fruits and vegetables: especially raisins, orange juice, potatoes, avocados, lima beans, tomatoes, apricots, or peaches.

Enjoy two to three servings a week of salmon, mackerel, sardines, or tuna, which contain omega-3 fatty acids (also available in capsule form) that help prevent or lower high blood pressure. It's better for you to substitute canola, safflower, or olive oils for saturated fats—this may cut your blood pressure by ten points.

A vegetarian diet can significantly reduce high blood pressure. If you do go "veggie," be sure to replace meats with vegetable protein: soy products, dried beans, nuts (go easy on them—they're fatty), seeds, and whole grains. Even if you don't go meatless, eat more fiber such as whole-grain breads, cereals, vegetables, and fruits.

Reduce animal fat, such as meat, eggs, butter, or cream. Eat more calcium, which is found in low-fat milk, yogurt, and cheese, along with sesame seeds, chickpeas, spinach, and broccoli. Also boost your magnesium intake by eating plenty of nuts, dried beans and peas, soybeans, dark green leafy vegetables, seafood, and low-fat milk.

Prevention

It's critical for you to have your blood pressure measured at least once a year. If you are overweight, start a weight-loss program and stick with it! Try on any of these aerobic exercises for size (twenty to thirty minutes a day, three times a week): jogging, bicycling, swimming, walking, aerobic dance, or tennis. Aerobic exercise lowers blood pressure when your pulse rate is raised and sustained for twenty minutes or longer. (Check with your physician before starting a weight-loss or exercise program.) Cut back (way back) on the salt to no more than 6 grams a day—and say no to fast food! Instead, cook with lemon juice, garlic, onions, herbs and spices to add rich, sharp, or spicy flavors. Read food labels carefully for high salt (sodium) content. Cut down on caffeine, and have no more than one drink of alcohol a day to keep your pressure low.

Avoid the people, places, and situations that get on your last nerve, if possible. Kick those cigarettes to the curb if you haven't already—it hikes your blood pressure and increases your risk of stroke.

Helen Blue, 46, of Philadelphia, Pennsylvania, improved not only her health, but her lifestyle with the help of a holistic healer. Blue had already lost 45 pounds by dropping beef, pork, and chicken from her diet and adopting a vegetarian regimen. Still she suffered from hypertension and severe headaches. Fueled by a desire to rid herself of hypertension medication, she sought alternative medicine. Her chiropractor, who also practiced reflexology and massage, encouraged her to give up fish and to eat more fruits and vegetables and soy foods. "He said I needed to order my mind to relax. I needed to do more to bring my body in balance."

So once a week, Blue receives deep-pressure body massage as soothing music or inspirational tapes play in the background. Hot steam packs follow, to relax problem areas. She also receives massage with warm oils to de-stress, and reflexology for the headache pain. Meditation has become a regular practice. So has marveling at her new blood pressure, which has dropped to normal, 120/80. "You get your muscles and organs to relax and accept the treatment [your healer] gives," she says. "I've seen a tremendous change in my health, but also in the way I live my life."

Impotence

Impotence is a potentially devastating condition that can have a profound effect on a man, both physically and psychologically.

Impotence is the consistent inability to attain or maintain an erection for satisfactory sexual intercourse. Physical causes of impotence include vascular disease, diabetes, atherosclerosis, certain medications, nicotine, alcohol, drugs, kidney disease, neurological disorders, trauma, cancer, or surgery. An abnormality in the following physical functions can also cause impotence: adequate blood inflow or nerve supply to the penis; venous trapping mechanism (in the normal penis, blood is trapped in the veins of the penis, causing erection), function of hypothalamus and pituitary glands (which oversee testosterone production); production of testosterone in the testicles; or difficulty in becoming aroused. Psychological causes include stress, anxiety, depression, and relationship problems. Impotence can bring emotional side effects such as depression, insecurity, and loss of self-esteem.

Statistics
An estimated 30 million men in the United States are affected by impotence. Because of the stigma attached to the disorder, the actual number could be even higher. Presumably, Black men have a higher incidence than Whites due to the high rates of hypertension, diabetes, prostate cancer, and vascular diseases.

Treatments

AROMATHERAPY
Essential oils of clary sage, sandalwood, and ylang ylang encourage relaxation and feelings of sensuality. You might try adding 2 drops of each to 4 teaspoons massage oil or to a warm bath.

CHINESE MEDICINE
Traditional belief is that too much anxiety brings energy stagnation in the liver, which can create impotence. Sextone and cibot root are often prescribed. You'll need to see a specialist for specific dosages.

HERBAL REMEDIES

Yohimbine, which comes from the bark of the West African yohimbe tree, is said to improve erections in some men. Yohimbine opens the surface blood vessels of the penis and stimulates the release of the hormone norepinephrine. If you experience side effects (increased heart rate, anxiety, insomnia, hypertension, nausea), lower the dosage and gradually increase to the amount prescribed by a specialist. *Ginkgo biloba* can also help if the problem is inadequate blood flow to the penis.

MASSAGE

Lovers: learn how to relax each other with massage. This will help to relieve the stress and anxiety often associated with the inability to sustain an erection. There are books that can guide you through the art of sensual massage. Consult your local library or bookstore or new age bookstore.

MIND-BODY

Moderate exercise helps you relax and gives you an energy boost, so get moving! It also stimulates sexuality and increases physical awareness. But don't overdo it—prolonged or extreme exercise can wear you out. Practice yoga or meditation, too: they are both great relaxers. If your relationship with your partner has been adversely affected by this problem, you need to try to open the channels of communication with him or her to work through issues that you both may have. In the meantime, express intimacy in other ways than intercourse such as holding hands, talking, touching, massage, or kissing.

NUTRITION AND DIET

You should avoid alcohol and caffeine because they constrict blood vessels and inhibit blood flow needed to achieve an erection. Also, zinc is crucial to producing testosterone—try taking supplements.

Prevention

Visit a urologist who will give you a complete physical examination, take blood tests to rule out treatable causes, and take a sexual and psychological history. Alcoholism, cocaine, crack, and marijuana are major causes of impotence. Just say no. Get your high blood pressure, elevated cholesterol, diabetes, and heart disease under control. See if any medications could be responsible. If you've had surgery, check with your doctor to see if you've experienced nerve or vascular damage that can be reversed.

Infertility

For many couples, the experience of trying to have a baby is complicated by infertility, which leads to great psychological stress, because the reasons are not always apparent. Infertility is the inability to conceive after having unprotected intercourse for one year or more. Infertility can be caused by inadequate production of healthy sperm, the failure to ovulate, a deformed uterus, blocked fallopian tubes, a hormonal imbalance (periods longer than six days, cycles shorter than twenty-four days or more than thirty-five days, very heavy periods), multiple miscarriages, environmental factors, sexually transmitted disease, trying to get pregnant in the late thirties (female fertility declines with age), heavy alcohol or cigarette consumption, certain prescription medications, exposure of female to DES (diethylstilbesterol—a synthetic hormone that was given to millions of women from 1941 to 1971 to prevent miscarriage, but that caused cancer and reproductive problems in their offspring) while in the mother's womb, exposure of male genitals to elevated temperatures. The medical risks for men include hernia repair, undescended testicles, a history of prostatitis (irritation/inflammation of the prostate gland), genital infections, and mumps after puberty. Infertility is successfully treated in more than 50 percent of couples after a year of treatment.

Statistics

As many as one in six American couples (more than 5 million people) experience some degree of infertility. African American couples are affected almost one and a half times more often than Whites.

Treatments

ACUPUNCTURE/CHINESE MEDICINE

Traditional Chinese medicine has been used to treat blocked fallopian tubes, endometriosis, amenorrhea (absence of menstrual cycle), and infertility related hormone problems. Talk to an Oriental medicine doctor about acupuncture and herbal treatments to address infertility issues.

FOLK REMEDIES

Although unproven, here are some down-home remedies. Use egg white as a vaginal lubricant to induce conception. Use only on the days during the month when the woman is fertile; and apply to the male's penis or her vagina. **Don't use if allergic to eggs.** Ladies, don't douche—it interferes with the pH level (acidity) of your vagina. Avoid caffeine in foods and drinks. Gentlemen, keep your testicles cool by avoiding excessive exercise, hot tubs, close-fitting underwear, and temperature extremes. Abstain from sex for two days prior to the woman's fertile time to let sperm build up, then have sex every other day. And when having sex, do it in the missionary position (man on top).

MIND-BODY

It's important to maintain a healthy weight. Being underweight or overweight can sometimes interfere with conception.

Don't overexercise—it can reduce sperm count and suppress ovulation. Chill way out; stress can affect the ability to conceive. You can try these techniques to de-stress, too: meditate, indulge in regular massage, acupressure, or aromatherapy, enjoy pleasant activities, take a walk, garden, visualize or listen to soothing music.

NUTRITION AND DIET

Eat lots of whole-grain cereals; fresh fruits and vegetables; lean protein; cooked dried beans and peas. Eat vegetable oils rather than animal fats. Increase vitamin E, found in wheat germ, nuts, vegetable oils, and seeds. Avoid alcohol and caffeine (they affect sperm production and ovulation). Zinc is also important to increase fertility—take a supplement of 15 milligrams a day along with 2 milligrams of copper. Vitamin C may improve sperm count—so, gentlemen, be sure to eat lots of citrus fruits or take a supplement (see label for dosage).

Prevention

Quit smoking and drinking (which affects sperm production and ovulation). Get a thorough medical examination before trying to conceive. Follow a healthy lifestyle. Rid your life of stress. Eliminate as many prescription medications as you can. Avoid vaginal lubricants (try egg whites instead, to increase sperm motility). Men, keep your testicles cool (heat kills sperm). Women, remain on your back for thirty minutes after sex. Don't worry too much about conceiving!

Excessive or very low body fat and chronic diseases such as diabetes, lupus, arthritis, hypertension, and asthma can affect ovulation and fertility—see a doctor. If your mother took DES when she was pregnant with you, tell your doctor so an x-ray can be done to assess the size and shape of your uterus. Avoid exposure to workplace hazards or toxins.

Insomnia

No one knows why we need sleep, but research has shown that it is essential for survival in both humans and animals. Insomnia is the inability to sleep or to remain asleep throughout the night. Transient (short-term) insomnia lasts up to three weeks; chronic insomnia persists for more than six weeks, usually for months or years. Symptoms include difficulty falling or staying asleep; early wakefulness; less total sleep time; and awaking unrefreshed. Insomnia often begins with a period of stress. Chronic sufferers show their tension in headaches, palpitations, cold hands or feet, or lower-back pain. Insomnia is caused by stress, anxiety, intestinal problems, heart disease, diabetes, anemia, yeast infections, chronic sinus infection, medications, and diet.

Statistics

Insomnia is very common, hitting about 20 percent of the population. Because the disorder is often stress-related, African Americans are especially susceptible.

Treatments

AROMATHERAPY
Lavender is considered a relaxing scent. Add a few drops to your bath water or buy an infuser and scent your bedroom with it to become more relaxed. Other relaxing oils include Roman chamomile, neroli, marjoram, or rose.

CHIROPRACTIC
In addition to relieving tension, chiropractors can help correct posture problems that contribute to sleeplessness.

FOLK REMEDY

No one has a sound scientific idea why warm milk helps some people sleep. One possible reason is that it is laced with the amino acid tryptophan and contains natural opiates thought to cause drowsiness.

HERBAL REMEDIES

Drink valerian or passionflower tea forty-five minutes before bedtime. Also try anise, celery seed, clove, cumin, fennel, garlic, ginger, honey, lime peel, marjoram, onion, orange peel, parsley, sage, spearmint, catnip, lady's slipper, chamomile, or skullcap in a tea. Drink thirty to forty-five minutes before bedtime for more restful nights.

MASSAGE

Stress is one of the leading causes of insomnia. You can manage your stress with regular massage, a major stress-reliever.

MIND-BODY

Progressive muscle relaxation, yoga, deep breathing, meditation, biofeedback, and cognitive focusing are effective relaxation techniques you can do yourself. Participate in aerobic exercise twenty to thirty minutes, three to five times a week—it will help release sleep-enhancing endorphins, which are body chemicals that give you a feeling of well-being. Don't exercise less than five to six hours before bedtime though; it can prevent your body temperature from falling and interfere with a good night's sleep.

NUTRITION AND DIET

The synthetic hormone melatonin is a sleep-regulating substance that can help reset the body's internal clock and markedly decrease insomnia and jet lag after extended air travel. See the label for dosage.

Make sure you're getting enough calcium (at least 800 milligrams a day) and magnesium (350 milligrams for men, 300 milligrams for women) daily. B-complex vitamins are helpful for good sleep. If you're eating regular, nutritious meals, you may be getting the full recommended dietary allowances in your food. If not, add a daily multivitamin. Tryptophan, found in milk and other dairy products, meats, rice, lima beans, and many proteins, is an amino acid that jump-starts the body's production of serotonin, the hormone that regulates sleep, appetite, mood, and pain. Another way to boost serotonin production in the brain is to eat carbohydrates (starches or sugars) several hours before bedtime.

Prevention

Getting a good night's sleep shouldn't be difficult if you follow these tips. Establish a regular bedtime and rising time; avoid physical exertion and mental stimulation just before sleep; don't go to bed too early; and avoid naps. Improve your sleep environment by sleeping on a firm mattress, dimming the lights, wearing loose-fitting clothing, and making sure there is good ventilation and the temperature is moderate. To promote sound sleeping, limit or avoid caffeine completely, especially after early afternoon; modify your alcohol consumption; stop smoking; exercise regularly; eliminate or lessen stress; and expose yourself to more sunlight.

Kidney Disease

Kidneys remove waste products from blood and regulate the balance of water and chemicals in the body. When they fail to function properly, waste products and excess fluids build up inside the body, causing a variety of symptoms including: swelling of the hands and feet, frequent thirst, shortness of breath, a frequent urge to urinate, the passing of a small amount of urine, puffiness around the eyes, an unpleasant taste in the mouth, a urine-like odor of the breath, chronic fatigue, increasingly high blood pressure, pale skin, and excessively dry and persistently itchy skin. If left untreated, the kidneys stop working altogether and dialysis or a kidney transplant is needed to clean the blood of waste products.

There are two types of kidney disease: acute (sudden loss of function) or chronic (gradual deterioration). Common causes of kidney disease include diabetes, high blood pressure, and atherosclerosis—all of which impede the flow of blood inside the kidneys. Lupus and other immune-system diseases that affect blood vessels may also inflame kidneys and trigger kidney disease. Some types of kidney disease are inherited or congenital. They can be caused by long-term exposure to toxic chemicals or drugs, or too much vitamin D or protein in diets of the elderly or the very ill.

Kidney stones are pebble-like crystals that sometimes form in kidneys. Sometimes they pass with pain through the ureter (tube connecting the kidneys to the bladder). Symptoms include back pain above the waist on one side of the body. Kidney disease is nothing to play around with: it can be life-threatening. Discuss any alternative treatments, especially herbal remedies, with your physician first.

Statistics

Twenty-nine percent of people treated for kidney failure are African Americans. Blacks ages twenty-four to forty-four are twenty times more likely than Whites to develop hypertension-related kidney failure.

Treatments

FOLK REMEDIES

Acidic beverages such as cranberry juice, vegetable juice cocktail, or vinegar diluted in water prevent or flush out calcium kidney stones. You also might try a concoction of baking soda and water to help dissolve uric acid and cystine stones.

HERBAL REMEDIES

Many herbs can be harmful in the treatment of kidney disease. Make sure you consult with a physician before using any herbal therapies. Here are a few suggestions for treating kidney stones you can try: Goldenrod tea can increase urine flow to help pass stones. Steep 2 teaspoons of flowers in two cups boiling water. Let stand twenty minutes, strain, and drink. Also good to try: put 3 teaspoons of dried stone root in 1 cup of water. Simmer fifteen minutes, drink three times a day. *Aloe vera* juice also helps reduce the size of kidney stones.

NUTRITION AND DIET

If you have kidney disease, restricting protein can delay or even prevent kidney deterioration, especially if your kidney disease is caused by diabetes. If you have diabetes, follow a diet that keeps your blood glucose levels within a tight range. A restricted diet (no more than 2 grams a day of potassium; 1 gram of protein per kilogram of body weight a day; 1 gram a day of phosphorus; 2 grams a day of sodium, in advanced cases) can keep body fluids and chemicals in balance, decrease the workload on diseased kidneys, and stop the buildup of waste products in the body. You should take calcium supplements to counteract bone weakening.

If you have kidney stones, lay off calcium-rich foods like milk, cheese, butter, and other dairy foods. Avoid foods rich in oxalate such as beans, beets, beer, celery, chocolate, grapes, green peppers, mustard greens, cocoa, or tea. Try a magnesium supplement or eat magnesium-rich foods such as whole-grain breads and cereals, soybeans, dark, green leafy vegetables, or seafood. Take vitamin B_6 to lower the amount of oxalate in urine. Go with vitamin A, it keeps the lining of the urinary tract healthy and helps discourage future stones from forming. Aim for 5,000 IU a day of vitamin A-rich foods (½ cup canned sweet potatoes has 7,982 IU). Other vitamin-rich foods include apricots, broccoli, cantaloupe, beef liver, and winter squash. Don't eat more than 6 ounces per day of protein-rich foods (too much protein favors kidney stones). As with other kidney diseases, cut down on salt (found in luncheon meats, chips, processed cheese, and pickled foods, for example). It's important to drink at least six to eight glasses of water daily—enough to urinate 2 quarts a day. Eat more vegetables and whole-grain cereals; reduce animal protein. Use extra virgin olive oil each day in cooking or salad dressings.

Prevention

Kidney disease has been linked to certain chemicals found in common household solvents, cleansers, and other products. Read labels carefully and avoid exposure to cadmium, carbon tetrachloride, chloroform, ethylene glycol, oxalic acid, tetrachloroethylene. Also, get moving! Activity pulls calcium away from your bloodstream (where it can help form kidney stones) and back into your bones where it belongs. Walking, running, swimming, or biking are great choices for healthy kidneys.

Liver Disease

Drinking excessive amounts of alcohol may give you more than a hangover—it can also damage your liver. The liver lies in the upper right side of your abdomen near the lower ribs. It is connected to the small intestine by the bile duct, which carries bile (a digestive fluid) formed in the liver to the intestines. It also regulates the metabolism of cholesterol, helps maintain normal blood sugar, helps blood clot, detoxifies drugs and poisons (including alcohol), and stores energy (glycogen) to fuel muscles.

Cirrhosis is a chronic liver disease where normal liver cells are damaged and replaced by scar tissue, decreasing the amount of normal liver tissue and eventually causing liver failure. Alcoholism (yes, it's a disease) is both a physical and psychological dependency on alcohol that can lead to cirrhosis. Other causes of cirrhosis include hepatitis B, C, or D; and inherited or congenital diseases. Symptoms include loss of appetite, nausea and vomiting, weight loss, enlarged liver, jaundice, itching, and vomiting of blood.

Gallstones are crystals that form when bile stored in the gall-bladder (a small, pear-shaped organ found underneath the liver) contains too much cholesterol. Gallstones are usually harmless and produce no symptoms, but they can cause irritation or even get stuck in the bile duct. Symptoms in mild cases include moderate pain in the upper part of the stomach and a bloated feeling. Symptoms in severe cases include intermittent pain in the upper right abdomen or between your shoulder blades, chronic indigestion, jaundice, and nausea. Here's what increases your risk: obesity, old age, being female, pregnancy, taking oral contraceptives, taking estrogen replacement therapy after menopause, heredity, or extreme weight loss over a short period of time.

Hepatitis is an inflammation of the liver that can be caused by a virus, alcohol, and some drugs. There are three types of viral hepatitis. Hepatitis A is caused by contact with a virus through contaminated food, water, or fecal matter inadvertently passed from hand to mouth. Hepatitis B is caused by a blood-borne virus transmitted sexually or through contaminated needles. Hepatitis C is transmitted through blood transfusions or infected needles. Symptoms of viral (also called infectious) hepatitis in the acute stage include fatigue, listlessness, jaundice, aches, nausea, and lack of appetite. In the chronic stage, hepatitis B and C can cause fatal liver failure.

Statistics
African Americans have the highest infection rate for hepatitis C and the second highest rate for hepatitis B of any other population group in the United States.

Treatments

ACUPUNCTURE/CHINESE MEDICINE

Acupuncture has been used in the treatment of hepatitis along with these herbs: wormwood and gardenia fruit. Small gallstones are said to dissolve with herbs such as lysimachia, pyrrosia leaf, and rhubarb. See a specialist for dosages.

HERBAL REMEDIES

To restore liver function consider this: Alcoholics are deficient in zinc, magnesium, niacin, vitamin B_{12}, all of which are supplied by dandelion. Put 3 teaspoons of dandelion root in 1 cup water and simmer for five minutes. Drink this three times a day. Also, add leaves to salad.

Kelp is a good source of all B vitamins. Goldenseal root and yellow dock have potassium. Gotu kola has magnesium. Silymarin, an antioxidant, is found in milk thistle. All of these may stimulate production of new liver cells in people with cirrhosis. Make an infusion by pouring one cup of boiling water on 1 teaspoon of bruised seeds and allow to stand for ten minutes.

To relieve mild gallstone symptoms: Drink strong peppermint tea three to four times a day or take 20 drops of an alcohol extract of peppermint in 3 ounces water up to four times a day. Drink gentian tea. Or combine peppermint leaves, chamomile flowers, gentian root, and fennel seeds and make a tea. Drink it thirty minutes before meals to help prevent gallbladder attacks.

MIND-BODY

For hepatitis, regular exercise minimizes fatty build up in the liver. Massage, biofeedback or relaxation techniques may also be helpful in relieving your pain.

NUTRITION AND DIET

For gallstones, eat beans, legumes, and vegetables. Bulk up on fiber. Reduce intake of all fats except olive oil. Skip fried foods. Drink no more than two units of alcohol a day: one unit is one beer, one drink of hard liquor, or one glass of wine. Eat more bran, especially oat bran. Drink six to eight glasses of water a day.

For hepatitis, give up alcohol altogether or until liver functions have been restored to normal. Moderation is the key. A high-fiber diet helps eliminate bile acids and toxic substances from your system. Avoid fried foods and animal fats. Limit simple carbohydrates (sugars and sweets) and saturated fats. Take vitamin C, vitamin B_{12}, and folic acid to shorten your recovery time.

Alfalfa detoxifies the liver and is a rich source of vitamins and other nutrients. Take in capsule or liquid form or enjoy alfalfa sprouts. Food allergies may contribute to gallstones. Under your physician's care, follow an elimination diet to determine what foods trigger them.

Prevention

Alcohol destroys liver cells, so avoid alcohol or don't drink to excess. Be cautious when using toxic chemicals at work, in the garden, or in housecleaning—make sure there's good ventilation, follow directions on products, avoid contact with skin, avoid inhaling chemicals, and wear protective clothing. To avoid gallstones, increase fiber, whole-grain cereals, fresh fruits and vegetables, oat bran, dried beans and peas. Reduce fat (especially saturated fat). A vegetarian diet helps prevent gallstones. Vaccines are available for hepatitis A and B, but to avoid the hepatitis virus, wash your hands with hot, soapy water after using the bathroom or changing diapers. And because hepatitis B can be transmitted sexually, be sure to practice safe sex (wear a condom or demand that your mate does). When traveling abroad, avoid dairy products, fresh fruits, and vegetables, and nonbottled water.

Lupus

Lupus, which literally means wolf in Latin, is a painful, and often-times debilitating disease that strikes African American women particularly hard. Lupus is a chronic autóimmune disease where the immune system loses its ability to tell normal connective tissues from foreign substances that enter the body and produces antibodies that attack normal tissues. This causes areas of the body to become inflamed, including joints, blood, skin, brain, lungs, kidneys, and heart. There are two types of lupus: DLE, or discoid lupus erythematosus, which affects skin exposed to sun; and SLE, or systemic lupus erythematosus, which is more serious and involves joints, the skin, brain, heart, kidneys, and other vital organs. There is no known cause for the disease; however, heredity, stress, too much sun, infections, hormonal changes and environmental factors may all play a role. High estrogen levels from hormone replacement, birth control pills, or pregnancy can trigger lupus. You can distinguish SLE from DLE because people with this type usually have a scaly, butterfly-shaped rash across the bridge of their nose and cheeks. Other general symptoms of lupus include fatigue, painful or swollen joints, purple or pale fingers or toes from poor circulation, unexplained chronic low-grade fevers, abdominal pain, unexplained weight loss or gain, sensitivity to the sun, hair loss, chest pain, nausea, low blood count, nose, mouth and throat sores, seizures, discolored urine, and frequent or blocked urination. What makes treatment so difficult for lupus is that symptoms appear, then leave, then come back, in no particular pattern.

Statistics

Of the 500,000 people with lupus in the United States, 90 percent are women, mostly ages fifteen to forty-five. Black women are three times as likely to develop lupus as White women.

Treatments

ACUPUNCTURE

Acupuncture may be helpful in treating symptoms. Seek out a qualified practitioner.

MIND-BODY

Although there is no cure for lupus, there are many alternative treatments you can try to deal with symptoms. However, don't stop taking prescribed medications, because lupus is a potentially fatal disease and your condition should be monitored by a physician. For example, attending a support group meeting will allow you to release emotions and share with others who know what you're going through. Meditation or yoga are also very helpful in combating stress. The human touch, in the form of acupressure or massage, can work wonders for swollen or tender joints.

NUTRITION AND DIET

Eating a nutritious diet is one key to staying healthy. You should also exercise, get plenty of rest, and don't smoke or drink.

Determine if you have any food allergies and avoid those foods. Avoid red meat and dairy products, and eat plenty of fish with omega-3 fatty acids (reduce inflammation), such as salmon or mackerel. Stay away from alfalfa—it makes symptoms worse. Get plenty of vitamin B_5, C, E, selenium, and slippery elm (check with a practitioner for dosage). For DLE, get plenty of beta-carotene (comes in carrots or squash and other yellow and orange vegetables).

Prevention

Keeping your body strong is essential to good health. Eat a wholesome diet, get lots of sleep, exercise, and avoid sun exposure or wear sunscreen. Also, keep stress at bay—you're better off in the long run.

Menopause

Menopause is a significant time in a woman's life that signifies the end of her fertile years. Menopause means literally, the end of menstruation. During a woman's fertile years, her ovaries produce hormones and an egg each month at ovulation. As menopause approaches, her egg production and menstrual periods become less regular until they stop altogether. These changes begin when the ovaries stop responding to sex hormones secreted by the pituitary gland. The resulting decline in the production of the female hormone estrogen causes the symptoms we associate with menopause. Menopause usually lasts four to five years and spans from two years before the last menstrual period to two to three years after, in women between ages forty-five to fifty-five.

Symptoms include heavier or lighter bleeding than normal, a period a day or two shorter or longer than normal before ceasing altogether, hot flashes (body heat and perspiration that come and go without warning), osteoporosis, vaginal dryness, vaginal pain or soreness during intercourse, pounding heartbeat, joint pains, headaches, itching skin, increased facial hair, mood swings, and depression.

Statistics

According to recent research, African American women begin menopause around age forty-nine, nearly two years before the onset of menopause in White women, who averaged fifty-one-and-a-half years. Smokers begin menopause even earlier.

Treatments

ACUPUNCTURE

Acupuncture is said to help reduce the frequency of hot flashes. Contact a specialist to develop a specific treatment regimen.

HERBAL REMEDIES

Ginseng is an herbal source of estrogen and is available as a tea. Black cohosh, dong quai, damiana, cramp bark, goldenseal, licorice root, oil of primrose, red raspberry leaves, sarsaparilla, and spearmint are also helpful. They're available in a dried form for tea and in capsules and powder.

HOMEOPATHY

By far, the most appropriate and effective remedy for menopausal symptoms is Sepia 6C (Cuttlefish). Another option would be Sanguina 6C (Blood Root), which has been found to be applicable to change-of-life disorders.

MIND-BODY

Relaxation techniques, biofeedback, visualization, hypnosis, meditation, and massage are helpful in managing hot flashes. Go with aerobic exercise three to four times a week, for twenty to thirty minutes to keep your body and mind in tip-top shape. Weight-bearing exercise protects against osteoporosis. Swimming for an hour three times per week has been shown to increase bone-mineral content. It also boosts your mood. Change your attitude about "the change": think of it as a natural process, not a disease.

NUTRITION AND DIET

As estrogen levels fall in menopausal women, calcium loss accelerates. Thus, postmenopausal women undergoing hormone replacement therapy need about 1,000 milligrams of calcium per day; women not receiving therapy need 1,500 milligrams per day.

Also, women going through menopause need to eat a diet rich in vegetables, fruits, complex carbohydrates, and nonfat or low-fat dairy products. Vitamin E may also help relieve hot flashes.

Hot drinks, hot meals, and spicy foods can aggravate hot flashes. So can sugar or simple refined carbohydrates (white flour, white rice, etc.) A vegetarian diet that excludes sugar can often help stop hot flashes promptly. Also avoid too much protein, salt and caffeine: All three substances can cause calcium loss. A very low-fat diet helps prevent osteoporosis as well as hot flashes. The following foods have plant sterols similar to estrogens. Eat plenty of them each day for natural estrogen replacement:

Fruits: apples, cherries, plums, coconut (though beware of coconut's calories and hard fats)

Whole grains: oats, rice, barley, corn, wheat, wheat germ

Herbs: parsley, anise seed, garlic, sage

Vegetables and nuts: carrots, yams, soybeans, and nightshade vegetables (bell peppers, eggplant, tomatoes, potatoes)

Vitamin E taken orally can be used to manage hot flashes. You can also puncture a vitamin E or vitamin A capsule and insert it as a vaginal suppository each night for vaginal dryness. Use daily for 6 weeks, then once or twice a week.

Make a tea from 1 teaspoon each of catnip, red raspberry leaf, alfalfa leaf, black cohosh, plus ¼ teaspoon licorice powder steeped in 3 cups boiling water. Take one cup, three times daily to relieve menopause symptoms.

Prevention

Avoid alcohol and caffeine, exercise regularly, and eat a healthful diet for the twenty years before menopause starts to avoid the need for hormone therapy. Wear loose clothing, keep your body temperature cool, use vaginal lubricants, begin calcium supplements at age thirty-five, don't smoke, and if you drink alcohol, do it in moderation.

Obesity

While some of us may "carry our weight well", we are putting ourselves at risk for disease or even death with severe weight gain. If you are obese, it means that your body fat is 30 percent or higher if you're a woman, and 25 percent or higher if you're a man. It also means you weigh 20 percent more than you should for your age, height, frame, and gender. Obese people burn calories faster and have a faster metabolism. Interestingly enough, one theory for the high rate of obesity among Blacks is that during the Middle Passage, only those captives who were able to effectively retain what they ate, survived. And before our ancestors were brought to the Americas, their diets consisted largely of fresh foods, which changed when they were fed the scraps of their slave-masters, changing their diet completely—for the worse. That legacy is now part of our "soul food" diet—the fried chicken, greens with ham hocks, lemon pound cake—you get the picture. These are all foods high in calories, sugar, and fat. Poverty plays a role, as well. Fresh produce may not be readily available or affordable and processed or fast foods high in calories and fat are substituted. Obesity is also caused by heredity, diabetes, metabolism, thyroid problems, some drugs (such as insulin or steroids), lack of exercise, and a bad diet (high calorie, high fat). The danger in obesity is that it puts you at higher risk for serious diseases such as colorectal cancer, coronary heart disease, diabetes, stroke, and hypertension, because that added girth strains the cardiovascular system and high amounts of fat can enlarge the liver.

Statistics
More than 30 percent of African Americans are overweight. About 45 percent of African American women are obese.

Treatments

ACUPRESSURE

If you seek out a practitioner, he or she might be able to help you control food cravings by pressing specific points on your ear.

CHINESE MEDICINE

If you seek out a practitioner, he or she might work on regulating your spleen and other vital organs to reduce food cravings.

HERBAL REMEDIES

If you want to speed up your metabolism, try kelp as a tablet. It's good for obese people with thyroid problems. To reduce food cravings, speed up metabolism, and keep kidneys clear, try dandelion leaves in a salad or as a tea: Boil 2 to 3 teaspoons of root in 1 cup of water for ten to fifteen minutes and drink three times a day. Cayenne and bee pollen may boost your metabolism.

HOMEOPATHY

If your obesity is related to overeating and excessive cravings for sweets, try Argentum Nitricum 6C (Nitrate of Silver); it works great for loss of control and lack of willpower.

MIND-BODY

Find ways to de-stress, such as yoga or guided imagery. Many Black women are stressed out from psychological overload, which is often attributed to poor self-image or physical or sexual abuse, and overeating is a way to feel better. Join a support group to find others who can share your weight loss goals. Get to stepping—power walking, that is—or swimming or biking. It will strengthen your heart, tone your body, and make you feel good as you burn those calories and fat and shed excess pounds. Make sure you stretch before and after working out to keep muscles limber. And no fitness routine is complete without some strength training component. **Check with your physician before starting an exercise plan.** Keep a food diary where you write down everything you eat and drink for a week. Make sure you note what time you're eating and how you are feeling when you're eating.

NUTRITION AND DIET

This is where you should start, because what you eat affects how much weight you gain or lose. Eat more fruits and vegetables, high quality proteins and complex carbohydrates. Ease up on the sugar, salty and fatty foods, alcohol, and dine on plenty of beans, vegetables, fruits and brown rice (these are low in fat and high in fiber). Opt for potatoes, pasta, fish, and chicken to fill up without it costing you. Also, put less food on your plate! While they sound promising, stay away from diet plans you may have heard of and wanted to try. You may actually end up gaining more weight because your body recognizes it's not getting enough to eat and slows down your metabolism and you ultimately put on more weight. Needless to say, this is not the desired effect. Instead, try eating your biggest meal at lunchtime when you burn more calories and two or three smaller meals throughout the day. Drink at least eight glasses of water a day.

Prevention

Avoid smoking (yes, it does make you less hungry but it also makes fat deposit around your waist) and excess drinking (it's processed like fatty foods). Eat a high-fiber, low-calorie, low-fat diet to help you reach your weight loss goals. And get moving!

Pregnancy and Childbirth

The wonder of the birth of a child brings plenty of joy and hope, but it can also wreak havoc on the mind and body of the mother.

Morning sickness usually occurs during the first trimester in some women, and can last until the second or third trimester. The symptoms include nausea and vomiting. Morning sickness is caused by the accumulation of estrogen and progesterone in the lining of the stomach while you sleep, which interact with the stomach acid and cause nausea in the morning, although it can occur at any time of day.

Nausea and constipation, which create significant discomfort, may be linked to increased levels of HCG (human chorionic gonadotropin, the pregnancy hormone) or changes in the digestive tract. Constipation is very common during pregnancy, especially during the last trimester. The placenta releases progesterone and stretches the uterine muscles so the baby can grow. Progesterone also slows muscle contractions so the fetus doesn't come out. However, the muscle of the intestine becomes less capable of moving the stool out. And during the last trimester, the uterus presses against the stomach and intestines because it's so large, which slows digestion and elimination.

Heartburn or indigestion is very common during pregnancy. Progesterone relaxes the muscle (esophageal sphincter) that closes the passage between the esophagus and stomach. This muscle allows food to enter the stomach when you eat. But if you're pregnant, some stomach acid flows up to the esophagus, causing a burning sensation.

Other common problems include fatigue, headaches, backache, leg, feet and ankle swelling, stretch marks, hemorrhoids and gum disease, which occur as a result of the pressure from the weight of the fetus and hormonal changes.

Despite the major changes that your body experiences, some women have reported that pregnancy offered an opportunity to embrace total wellness—eating well, not drinking alcohol and bonding with their unborn child.

Statistics

Heartburn affects 30 to 70 percent of pregnant women during the second and third trimesters. There is a higher incidence of low birthweight babies among African Americans, which contributes to a higher infant mortality rate.

Treatments

AROMATHERAPY

To make stretch marks disappear, add 20 drops of oil of mandarin orange and 5 drops jasmine to 4 ounces carrier oil and apply every day after your shower. Soak a cloth in cool water and add several drops of lavender for a headache or morning sickness. For digestion, massage your stomach with two drops each of peppermint and sandalwood mixed with 2 teaspoons carrier oil.

HERBAL REMEDIES

Ginger (taken as a tea or lozenge) helps relieve nausea caused by morning sickness. Mint or ginger tea helps relieve indigestion. To keep your uterus healthy, try red raspberry (strengthens uterus and reproductive system), and black and blue cohosh (stimulates uterine muscles during childbirth) teas to help ensure a problem-free labor and delivery. Chamomile tea helps with digestion and keeps you calm. Anise, catnip, fennel, and peppermint as teas are also good for morning sickness.

HOMEOPATHY

For morning sickness ask a homeopath about Colchium autumnale, Tabacum, or nux vomica.

MIND-BODY

Take it easy—stress is harmful to you and your unborn baby. Try massage, guided imagery, yoga, meditation, or moderate exercise. Look into yoga or exercise classes specifically designed for pregnant women. Exercise can also help keep your uterus healthy, and toning and light stretching will keep your abdominal muscles strong. If you exercised regularly before getting pregnant, keep it up (some women continue working out through their third trimester). If you didn't have an exercise program, after you get pregnant is not the time to launch into a rigorous fitness plan. Wear loose-fitting clothing to help prevent indigestion. For swollen feet and legs, try alternating cold and hot foot baths: Soak in hot water for three minutes, then in cold water for thirty seconds. Repeat this three to six times every day. For backaches, take a shower for sixty seconds in hot water, then a cold shower for thirty seconds, alternating three times, ending with the cold shower twice a day. Also, get plenty of rest to combat fatigue and stress. For hemorrhoids, try a warm sitz bath or apply cloth soaked in witch hazel.

NUTRITION AND DIET

Before getting pregnant, make sure you begin taking a good multivitamin with a high dosage of folic acid, which has been shown to reduce birth defects in newborns. Also, don't believe the hype: you can't give in to all those cravings and eat everything in sight. Watch what you eat—only a certain amount of those pounds will fall right off. To combat morning sickness, eat crackers or dry toast when you wake up, eat smaller, more frequent meals, avoid greasy, fried or spicy foods, and drink liquids after meals. Eating foods rich in vitamin B_6 such as bananas, walnuts, and wheat germ can alleviate symptoms. To keep your bowels moving, avoid cheese, chocolate, white rice, and bread. Try prunes, raisins, or apricots, eat more fiber, eat at regular mealtimes, and drink more liquids. For indigestion, eat smaller, more frequent meals, eat a high-fiber and protein, low-fat diet, eat slowly and chew your food well, avoid spicy, greasy, sugar-laden foods, and don't lie down after eating. For headaches, eat regularly and drink at least six glasses of water a day. Bulk up on fiber to avoid painful hemorrhoids and drink plenty of liquids. You can try taking supplements of vitamin C and calcium for gum disease. Consult your physician before incorporating any major vitamin program.

Prevention

Avoid coffee and alcohol while pregnant and breastfeeding. Alcohol can cause permanent damage to the fetus, such as fetal alcohol syndrome. Alleviate stress, which can affect the length of your pregnancy and your newborn's birthweight. Make sure you have good prenatal care from a medical practitioner and follow up with visits during pregnancy and after delivery. Eat a healthy diet and get regular, moderate exercise.

Prostate Problems

Prostate problems refer to any of several disorders that affect the prostate, which is a solid, walnut-shaped organ situated in front of a man's rectum and just below his bladder. The main function of the prostate is to produce seminal fluid, which protects sperm from the acidic environment inside the vagina. The gland is divided into the inner area (which can undergo benign enlargement, called benign prostatic hyperplasia [BPH]) and the outer area, which surrounds the urethra (the usual site of cancer formation). BPH is considered a normal consequence of aging. By the time men reach age sixty-five, about half of all men in the United States will have symptoms of BPH. They include difficulty, pain, increased frequency of or increased urgency in urination, or a combination of these symptoms.

Prostatitis, another common prostate condition, is an infection or inflammation that causes a man to experience pain in the genitals, lower pelvis or back. It does not lead to cancer nor is it connected to BPH.

Prostate cancer is known as the silent killer because it can occur without any symptoms. By the time a man experiences symptoms, the cancer is likely to be at an advanced stage. Some of the symptoms of prostate cancer include weak or interrupted urine flow, inability to urinate, or difficulty stopping or starting the flow.

Statistics

Prostate cancer is the most common cancer in African American men, and the second most common cause of cancer death (after lung cancer) in American men. One in eleven White men and one in nine Black men over age fifty will develop prostate cancer. While White men are urged to begin having regular prostate exams at fifty, Black men are encouraged to monitor their prostate with exams beginning at age forty.

Treatments

CHIROPRACTIC

Adjustments may assist in relieving back pain sometimes associated with prostatitis.

HERBAL REMEDIES

Two of the most common herbs used for prostate problems come from "home"—down South and the Motherland. Saw palmetto berries are said to help reduce prostate enlargement, therefore helping with symptoms from BPH.

African Pygeum, the bark from the African evergreen tree, is said to help control hormones that can cause prostate flare-ups. You can often find these two herbs blended in extract or capsule form. And the herbs have few, if any, side effects. Studies of the effects of herbs and supplements for prostatitis or prostate cancer have not been as revealing.

MIND-BODY

It's important to manage your stress with yoga, massage, visualization, deep breathing, or meditation. Also, get adequate sleep.

Exercise at least three to five days per week for twenty to thirty minutes.

NUTRITION AND DIET

You need to decrease the amount of fat and meat in your diet because there is evidence that high-meat, high-fat diets can increase the risk of prostate cancer. Increase the amount of fiber in your diet (about 50 to 100 grams per day), drink eight to ten glasses of water each day, and a good variety of fruit juices. Cranberry and raspberry juices are considered particularly helpful to the bladder and prostate. Zinc, found in lean meat and whole-grain breads, is considered essential for the normal growth, development, and functioning of the prostate gland. Antioxidants such as vitamin C, selenium, and beta-carotene are considered important in any anticancer diet. Vitamin C is prevalent in citrus fruits, green leafy vegetables, and green peppers. Indulge in them!

Because prostatitis is an infection, use herbs and vitamins with immune-enhancing or antibacterial properties like vitamin C, zinc, vitamin E, beta-carotene and others.

Prevention

Some studies indicate that tomatoes can help to reduce the risk of prostate cancer. While you're enjoying spaghetti and salsa, get a routine screening once a year for prostate cancer if you're an African American man over age forty. It involves a digital rectal examination and a blood test for prostate-specific antigen (PSA), a blood protein often present in cases of cancer. The test is simple, virtually painless, and inexpensive. While there are no definitive methods of preventing prostate cancer, taking control of your health—which includes following proper nutritional guidelines, exercising, managing stress, and educating yourself—is a major factor in living long and living well.

Sexually Transmitted Diseases

In this day and age, if you're sexually active, your life depends on protecting yourself from acquired immune deficiency syndrome (AIDS) and other sexually transmitted diseases (STDs), which can kill or stay with you for the rest of your life. STDs are infections transmitted through sexual intercourse, including AIDS, chlamydia, genital herpes, genital warts and hepatitis B (see liver disease for more information), gonorrhea, and syphilis. Because these are serious infections, antibiotics are usually prescribed. Antiviral drugs can prolong life for AIDS patients.

Statistics
Blacks account for about 80 percent of all reported cases of gonorrhea, and 46 percent of reported cases of syphilis. Black men are less likely than White men to receive medications that effectively treat human immunodeficiency virus (HIV) and prevent fatal infections that often complicate HIV. AIDS is the leading cause of death for blacks between the ages of twenty-five and forty-four. In fact, observers predict that in the next century, over half the national HIV-positive population will be Black.

Treatments

ACUPUNCTURE/CHINESE MEDICINE
Chinese herbs and acupuncture have proven to be highly effective in treating symptoms of AIDS, such as night sweats, fatigue, neuropathy, diarrhea and in relieving side effects of pharmaceutical drugs and radiation. Herbal remedies include ginseng, astragalus, ganodermam salvia, millettia, peony, gentiana, Chinese foxglove root, dong quai, and licorice. These are said to help cleanse the system. See a specialist for dosages.

HERBAL REMEDIES

For AIDS, goldenseal increases immunity and combats fungal infections (take as a tincture, consult a practitioner for dosage); garlic has antibacterial and antiviral properties.

For syphilis, add 2 tablespoons each of sarsaparilla and sourdock root to 1 quart boiling water. Simmer for five minutes and add 3 teaspoons thyme. Steep covered for one hour. Drink one to three cups a day.

For gonorrhea, try calendula, myrrh, and thuja in a tea or douche to reduce inflammation and discharge (for calendula tea, add 1 to 2 teaspoons petals to 1 cup of water twice a day). Calendula is also good as an ointment for herpes sores.

For chlamydia and genital infections, saw palmetto stimulates your immune system (drink in tea or take in capsules).

MIND-BODY

During an attack of genital herpes, take warm baths with 3 tablespoons table salt added. Take warm baths to also relieve pain from gonorrhea. For AIDS patients, meditation and massage will help ease stress, alleviate pain and muscle tension. Exercise also relieves stress.

NUTRITION AND DIET

To reduce occurrences of herpes attacks, reduce your intake of the amino acid arginine, which is found in nuts, chocolate, oats, coconut, whole-grain and white flour, wheat germ, and soybeans. Increase your intake of the amino acid lysine, which is found in fish, shrimp, chicken, milk, beans, brewer's yeast, fruits, and vegetables. Take 1 gram vitamin C with bioflavonoids every day during attacks. Follow a low-fat, high-fiber, and nutritious diet.

For chlamydia, eat whole-foods with a lot of protein, fruits, vegetables, and live yogurt with *Lactobacillus acidophilus.* Supplement with vitamin E and zinc.

For AIDS, follow a nutritious diet low in fat, sugars, refined, and convenience foods; high in fruits, vegetables, whole-grain breads and cereals, lean meats, cooked dried beans and peas, dairy, chicken, and fish. Take a multivitamin mineral supplement daily. Also, increase beta-carotene (found in green, leafy vegetables, orange, and yellow vegetables), vitamin C (stimulates immunity and is an antiviral), bioflavonoids (found in green, leafy vegetables, pith and rind of citrus fruits), and zinc (stimulates immunity and is an antiviral, 15 milligrams a day).

Prevention
Limit your number of sexual partners, practice safe sex, and always use a condom. Avoid having sex with anyone with a rash or discharge. Get regular Pap smears. Intravenous drug users should not share needles. Avoid alcohol and tobacco. Avoid sharing towels or clothing. Get a hepatitis B vaccine. Stay away from alcohol, nicotine, and recreational drugs that affect sperm production and ovulation.

Sickle Cell Disease

Sickle cell disease is an inherited, chronic blood disease in which the red blood cells become crescent or sickle shaped and function abnormally. This hereditary blood disease results when the oxygen-carrying protein, hemoglobin, is defective in red blood cells. These abnormal red blood cells lose the normal round contour and form a sickle shape that blocks blood vessels and the normal flow of oxygen in the blood. While sickle cell disease has been part of life in Africa for centuries, it also affects millions of people worldwide and is prevalent in South America, Cuba, Central America, Saudi Arabia, India, and Mediterranean countries including Turkey, Greece, and Italy. For reasons that doctors are still unclear about, the vast majority of people with sickle cell anemia are African-

Americans. An estimated 1 in 12 African-Americans carries the sickle cell trait, which is not the same as having the disease. However, carrying the trait increases the possibility of passing the trait and/or the disease to your children, especially if two people with the trait decide to have children together. In the United States, about 1,000 babies a year are born with sickle cell anemia.

Recurring episodes of excruciating pain called sickle cell "crises" are the most obvious symptom of the disease. Infants usually show symptoms of the disease after four months of age. If your baby has any of the following symptoms, contact a doctor immediately: fever, jaundice, swollen extremities and joints, or pneumonia.

Signs and symptoms in children and adults include: anemia, fatigue, frequent infections, painful joints, acute chest or abdominal pain, slow growth, leg ulcers, and stroke.

Although there is currently no cure for sickle cell disease, there are a number of treatments that can alleviate some of the pain associated with it. While it's not available to all sickle cell patients, Hydroxurea appears to be a promising drug that aids some patients by helping to prevent the sickling of red blood cells.

In the United States, the disease affects more than 70,000 people, predominantly African-Americans, according to the National Heart, Lung, and Blood Institute (NHLBI) of the National Institute of Health. Sickle cell disease occurs in about 1 of every 500 African-American births and 1 in every 1,000 to 1,400 Hispanic-American births. About 1 in 12 African-Americans carries the sickle cell trait.

Treatments

No cure is available for sickle cell disease. The objective of therapy is to manage and control the symptoms relating to crises.

AROMATHERAPY

Stress should be avoided as much as possible. Certain relaxation-inducing scents should be introduced into your home and work environments. Try lavender, Roman chamomile, marjoram, lemon-scented eucalyptus, and lemon balm.

MIND/BODY

Make sure you're getting enough sleep. Bed rest is critical during a crisis so that you avoid overexerting yourself. Drink plenty of fluids. Dehydration can make painful crises worse. Parents should encourage their children to lead normal lives. In order to decrease the occurrence of sickle cell crises, the following precautions should be considered:

- Avoid strenuous physical activity, especially if the spleen in enlarged

- Avoid emotional stress

- Avoid environments of low oxygen content (high altitudes, non-pressurized airplane flights)

- Avoid known sources of infection

- Recognize signs of dehydration

- Avoid excess exposure to the sun

- Provide access to fluids at home and away from home

- Keep your child properly immunized as recommended by your health care provider

- Consider having your child wear a Medic Alert Bracelet

- Share medical information with teachers and other caretakers as necessary

- Be aware of the effects that chronic, life-threatening illnesses can have on siblings, your marriage, parents, and the child

NUTRITION AND DIET

In chef Dawud Ujamaa's book *Back to Our Roots: Cooking for Control of Sickle Cell Anemia and Cancer Prevention*, he asserts that diet is a key factor in the control of sickle cell disease. The book is based on the fact that although an estimated 25 percent of people in Africa carry the sickle cell trait, very few cases of sickle cell anemia are reported. Diet is believed to be the key. Several foods that are part of the African diet are rich in cyanates, which are known to stop sickling. (Cyanates are a nontoxic relative to the poison cyanide.) Foods such as buckwheat, cassava, garbanzo beans, lentils, millet, sorghum, and the African yam all contain nutritional cyanate. Other more familiar cyanate-rich foods include mustard greens, lima beans, bananas, cabbage, and other fruits and vegetables.

Folic acid supplementation is also used for continuous therapy.

Prevention

Genetic counseling is recommended for carriers of the sickle cell trait. Prompt treatment of infections, adequate oxygenation, and drinking plenty of fluids may prevent sickling of red blood cells. Prenatal diagnosis is also possible for couples at risk of producing a child with sickle cell anemia. For more information call the Sickle Cell Disease Association of America, 200 Corporate Pointe, Suite 495, Culver City, CA 90230; 1-800-421-8453.

Skin Problems

Acne is usually associated with the teenage years; however, it can occur in adulthood, along with a range of other skin problems. Acne refers to pimples, blackheads, or whiteheads on the face, neck, or back due to hormonal changes that lead to an increase in oily skin and clogged pores.

Eczema is an inflammation of the skin usually in the creases of elbows, knees, and armpits, with itching, redness, blisters, scales or scabs. Eczema is caused by dietary problems, emotional stress, chemical irritants, or allergies.

Psoriasis is characterized by thick, red patches covered by a silvery scale, usually around the elbows, knees, scalp, trunk, and back. It tends to run in families.

Keloids are smooth, thick, elevated scars that appear on the skin after a burn, cut, or other trauma. Keloids can be painful and often run in families.

Pseudofolliculitis, or razor bumps, are pimplelike swellings caused when sharp, coarse hairs curl back into the skin. Razor bumps can cause painful irritation and infection.

Statistics

Keloids are extremely common among African Americans of both sexes. Razor bumps are special problems for African American men. Whereas White men's facial hair tends to grow out straight, Black men's facial hair grows out and then curls into a ball with the already sharp shaven edge pointing into the skin.

Treatments

AROMATHERAPY

Bathe daily in warm water with 2 drops essential oil of lavender added for acne.

CHINESE MEDICINE

Practitioners use Oriental wormwood, Chinese gentian, peony root, or rumania for eczema. See a specialist for dosage. For acne, they use cnidium seed topically and honeysuckle flower to clear damp heat on the skin and kill parasites.

HERBAL REMEDIES

For acne, add 1 teaspoon dried Blue flag herb to 1 cup water. Simmer ten minutes. Drink three times a day to rid your body of toxins.

For eczema, try evening primrose oil to relieve itching.

For psoriasis, try burdock for dry, scaly skin: Add 1 teaspoon root to 1 cup water. Simmer fifteen minutes. Drink three times a day.

For keloids, rub *Aloe vera* on the affected area.

HOMEOPATHY

To address the wide range of skin problems using homeopathic remedies, here is a list of options:

- Calcarea Silicata 6C (Silicate of Lime)—to clear acne

- Kali Bichromicum 6C (Bichromate of Potash)—for itchy spots

- Sulphur 6C (Sulphur)—for red, sore infected spots or eczema

- Graphites 6C (Black Lead)—used for burning, hot itchy skin

- Petroleum 6C (Crude Rock Oil)—when skin is cracked and oozing

MIND-BODY

Get plenty of exercise to alleviate stress, which can trigger eczema. Aerobic exercise opens pores, allowing your skin to breathe. Try some physical activity for thirty minutes, three times a week.

NUTRITION AND DIET

For acne, avoid fats, sugars, refined foods and junk foods. Eat lots of raw fruits and vegetables, whole-grain breads and cereals, cooked dried beans, low-fat dairy products, chicken, and fish. Increase: zinc (found in poultry, fish, organ meats, whole-grain breads, cereals, or take as a supplement).

For eczema, increase vitamin A (found in egg yolk, liver, kidney, butter, whole milk, cod liver oil) and niacin (found in lean meat, fish, cooked, dried beans and peas, peanut butter); take vitamin B complex; rid your diet of potential food allergens such as dairy products, wheat, corn, soybeans, food and drink preservatives, colorants, additives; replace cow's milk with goat's milk or soy milk; for inflammation, take vitamin C and bioflavonoids as supplements or in citrus fruits. For psoriasis, reduce meat, animal fats, sugar, and alcohol. Increase fiber, fish, fruits, vegetables, wholegrain cereals, cooked dried beans and peas. Take linseed oil, zinc, vitamin B complex, vitamin A. Be cautious of possible allergies to dairy products and citrus fruits.

Prevention

For acne, avoid oil-based cosmetics. Try not to touch your face with your hands, which carry dirt and bacteria and can clog pores. Wash your skin well with soap or nonirritating cleanser. Don't squeeze pimples or whiteheads; it can cause scarring.

For eczema, avoid harsh detergents and soaps; be cautious about aggravating affected area by wearing jewelry or bra straps; and wear plastic or cotton gloves for household and garden work.

For keloids, avoid injuring the skin with costume jewelry and razor shaves.

For razor bumps, use a double blade and shave in the direction hair grows, or use a depilatory cream. Use a steamy towel to soften your beard before shaving. Don't shave too close—the closer the shave, the more likely you'll get razor bumps. Use a clean sharp blade. The only foolproof technique is to avoid shaving completely.

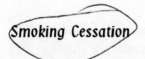

Smoking Cessation

It's a wonder anyone smokes, with all the publicity about how bad tobacco is for you. Lungs filled with tobacco smoke can surely lead to heart disease, emphysema, chronic bronchitis, and a host of other debilitating and sometimes fatal illnesses—not to mention cancer of the lung, larynx, esophagus, uterus, ovaries, cervix, kidney, pancreas, and bladder. It's the nicotine in tobacco smoke that keeps smokers hooked with a vengeance that experts say is more severe than heroin addiction. But there is hope if you're serious about taking that last puff.

Statistics

Smoking is often a response to stress, and African Americans are subjected to mega-stresses each and every day. About 5 million of the 46 million adult smokers in the United States are African Americans. About 26 percent of Blacks smoke as compared with 25.4 percent of Whites. Lung cancer is the leading cause of cancer death among Blacks, but our children may change that statistic one day: only 20 percent of young Black males (versus 30 percent of White males) and 8 percent of young Black females (versus 27 percent of White females) are smokers.

Treatments

ACUPUNCTURE

Acupuncture reduces withdrawal symptoms by increasing willpower and relieving tension, depression, anxiety, insomnia, cravings, body aches, headache, and nausea. It releases endorphins to make the body more resistant and eliminates harmful chemicals in the body while eliciting relaxation. Seek out a qualified practitioner and get to work.

HERBAL REMEDIES

Lobelia and nicotine have similar effects on the body. Lobelia can be extremely toxic, so take it only under the direction of a naturopath or homeopath. It is sold in tablets, lozenges, or chewing gum to help minimize the discomfort of withdrawal symptoms. Take ginseng as a tea or in capsules. Try valerian tea for its calming effect.

HOMEOPATHY

Talk to a homeopath about Allertox Tobacco, which is said to relieve nicotine cravings.

MIND-BODY

Choose an affirmation (a positive statement, like "I'm feeling relaxed" or "I'm in control"). It helps remind you why you are no longer smoking and imprints an image of health in your mind that your body can emulate. Repeat this affirmation when you feel a craving coming on (they typically last two minutes). In case this doesn't offer immediate relief, have a Plan B—breathe deeply, take a walk somewhere, sing a song, dance, call a friend. Support groups can be extremely helpful, especially during initial attempts to quit, which can be challenging. Hypnosis has also proven to be an effective route to smoking cessation.

Hydrotherapy is another creative option that can help you detoxify your body while trying to kick the habit. It goes like this: Take a hot shower, wrap your body in a sheet (refer to page 87 for a full description).

NUTRITION AND DIET

To help pull you through those difficult first few weeks after quitting, drink lots of citrus juice or take 1,000 milligrams a day of vitamin C supplements. Sip water frequently throughout the day: dryness causes cravings. Also, cut out the coffee—it causes cravings and dehydration. Eat a lot of carrots, celery, and other vegetables instead of candy, which upsets blood-sugar levels and can aggravate nicotine-withdrawal symptoms. Eat six daily meals of fresh fruits, vegetables, proteins, whole-grain breads, and pasta. This combination keeps blood-sugar levels steady and helps to prevent the food cravings that often mess with smokers during nicotine withdrawal.

Prevention
If you do smoke, try not to do it around your children. Studies have proven that there is an increased likelihood that they too will become smokers. Eat a balanced, nutritious diet; avoid stressful situations and people; involve yourself in activities you enjoy; get plenty of rest; slow down and take a deep breath. Avoid alcohol.

Stress

If there's one thing African Americans are used to, it's stress. We are confronted with this every day on our jobs, in our communities, and at home. Stress is defined as a constant state of tense alertness. The body responds to stressors, whether short or long-term, by tensing muscles and constricting blood vessels in a natural "fight or flight" reaction. Since the 1980s, the medical community has begun to acknowledge the link between stress and diabetes, hypertension, heart attacks, and other common ailments that plague African Americans. Chronic (prolonged) stress can also weaken the immune system. Symptoms include headaches; dizziness; rash; colds and infections; anxiety; sexual problems; heart palpitations; high blood pressure; fatigue; pain in the neck, shoulders, or back; loss of appetite; compulsive eating; sleep problems; irritability; and difficulty concentrating.

Statistics
Racism and poverty subject African Americans to significantly more chronic stress than Whites. African American men die from heart disease at a rate 47 percent higher than White men, partly because of the effects of stress on the cardiovascular system. Hyper-

tension, closely linked to stress, affects one in four African Americans and one in six Whites.

Treatments

ACUPUNCTURE/CHINESE MEDICINE

Acupuncture can induce deep relaxation. There are also several Chinese herbs considered good for stress relief: thorowax root, peony root, schizandra fruit. See a specialist for dosages.

AROMATHERAPY

This is sure to relax you: To a nice, warm bath add five to six drops essential oil of lavender. Or put two to three drops on a handkerchief and inhale to promote relaxation. Other oils to try include Roman chamomile, marjoram, lemon-scented eucalyptus, and lemon balm.

HERBAL REMEDIES

Try a cup of chamomile, passion flower, valerian or American ginseng tea to take your cares away.

MASSAGE

Massage is good for relieving tense muscles, aching backs, shoulders, and headaches. It also improves your blood circulation and relaxes your mind.

MIND-BODY

Aerobic exercise helps relax the mind and body and stimulates a sense of well-being. Try one of these for at least thirty minutes, three times a week: running, walking, cycling, swimming, aerobics. Meditation takes you into a deep state of relaxation. Saying self-affirmations, visualization, and deep-breathing exercises help, too.

NUTRITION AND DIET

The human body isn't built to absorb junk foods and foods with highly refined sugar. Too many sweets can actually contribute to low blood sugar, which is a stress on the system. Too much caffeine can also lead to a shaky feeling and aggressiveness. Eat food naturally rich in vitamins, such as carrots, greens, and other vegetables and fruits. Eat lots of whole-grain breads and cereals.

Prevention

To keep stress to a minimum, eat a balanced, nutritious diet and avoid stressful situations and people, if possible. Involve yourself in activities you enjoy; get plenty of rest; and slow down and take a deep breath. Avoid alcohol and caffeine, which can make you anxious and jittery.

The Healing Power of Baths (by K. Anna Monsho)

When I was a girlchild, my grandmother, who we called Bigmama, always told me that cleanliness is next to godliness. "Babygirl," she'd say in her honeyed Alabama whisper. "Something about water and the Spirit, they just naturally go together." It wasn't until I was a woman that I realized immersing in a tub of warm fragrant water could put me in touch with my soul life. Instead of focusing on getting clean, my bath has become a ritual for getting clear.

Today's health wisdom says bathing's benefits go beyond relaxation. Immersion in a bath is one type of treatment in a healing method called hydrotherapy—water therapy—that uses different intensities and methods of applying water. It includes not only bathing, but also showers, douches, sitz baths, and the application of friction and steam.

"Hydrotherapy is something naturopaths have been using for years," says Andrea Sullivan, N.D., a naturopathic doctor based in Washington, D.C. The theory behind this healing method is that using different temperatures of water to change the temperature of the body has a healing effect.

Hydrotherapy claims ancient origins, and many cultures still use it as part of the healing process.

"Hippocrates was the first person to use hydrotherapy," Dr. Sullivan says. The ancient Egyptians added botanicals, salts, and aromatic oils to bath water from the Nile, which was thought to remove negative energy associated with ill health. Legend has it that Cleopatra added honey and the milk of an ass to her bath to enhance her beauty. On this continent, Native Americans participate in sweat lodge ceremonies—closing themselves in a dark, sauna-like hut—as part of a powerful spiritual cleansing ritual.

Atlanta, Georgia-based herbalist and naturopath, Dr. Stephen Tates, has been prescribing herbal baths to his clients for over twenty years. He says that herbal baths can help reduce stress, flush impurities from the body, soothe skin conditions, and otherwise nourish the body.

"Properties of nutritional herbs are absorbed through the skin and act as a tonic," he says. "Circulation is assisted by using mint, cayenne, and ginger, and stress is lessened by using lavender, hops, and chamomile."

Dr. Sullivan recommends adding Dead Sea salt to your bath, especially for muscle aches. "It acts as an astringent. It literally draws toxins out of the body," she says.

Dr. Tates feels strongly about the necessity of using water for health, both internally and externally. He says, "You can get all the exercise and vitamins and herbs in the world, but if you are not consciously drinking enough water and taking therapeutic baths, at least occasionally, you are shortchanging your body."

Michelle Bibby is sure to get her fair share of bathing's benefits.

"I try to have a bath every day," says Bibby, who facilitates empowerment workshops for African Americans in Austin, Texas. "I use candles, put on some gospel music, and pour in bath salts. Atmosphere is important, and the aroma is completely relaxing."

She knows what she's talking about. Aromatherapy uses the essential oils of plants and flowers to alter mood and neutralize stress. Scent immediately affects the brain in a way that nothing else can, affecting the limbic and hypothalamus areas that in turn control mood, memory, intuition, sex drive, and emotion, aromatherapists say.

Aromatherapy invokes a powerful healing response when combined with hydrotherapy. It's especially effective in baths where the combination of heat and relaxation enhance absorption.

It wasn't healing that Cynthia Polk-Allen was looking for when she first started taking baths: it was peace of mind. A mother of two small girls, she works full time as a marketing director for a major bank in Manhattan and attends school to study natural healing. In her hectic life, Polk-Allen says her baths are her salvation.

"I have to keep my life in balance. My bath keeps me sane," she explains. "It's the one time when I can get away from deadlines, demands, and the hustle and bustle just to spend time healing myself." She has learned that adding rosemary and bay leaves to her bath makes all the difference in the world in how she feels when she emerges.

My grandmother was right. The bath ritual is a way to honor and heal ourselves—body, mind and spirit. In a meditative bath, with the help of hot water, bath oil, candlelight, and music, I find peace. I emerge relaxed, feeling and smelling divine, in touch with life, ready to face the world or sleep peacefully through the night.

Varicose Veins

One folk remedy for varicose veins that works: wearing support socks or pantyhose. If you're a varicose vein sufferer, you'll want to read on.

Varicose veins, which look like the blue or red lines on a map running down your arms or legs, occur when veins become less elastic and weaken, developing clots and swelling. Symptoms include sore, achy, tender legs; deep blue blood vessels under skin in legs and feet; thick, bulging blue veins; swollen feet and ankles; discolored, peeling skin; and skin sores. Varicose veins can be inherited and can result from intense pressure on the veins in the legs or abdomen from obesity, pregnancy, prolonged sitting, old age, or constipation.

Statistics

More than 20 million people, or nearly 10 percent of men in the United States and 20 percent of women, have varicose veins.

Treatments

AROMATHERAPY

To help relieve pain and swelling, massage oil of rosemary, cypress, or chamomile around the sore area (stimulates circulation). Try this concoction: Blend 12 drops each of oil of cypress and geranium with 4 ounces carrier oil and gently stroke upward around the sore area and massage on veins.

CHIROPRACTIC

A practitioner might advise you about your diet and use manipulation to alleviate pain caused by pressure on the pelvis; manipulation will also improve circulation.

HERBAL REMEDIES

Try butcher's broom (as an ointment, tincture, or tea) or horse chestnut (as an ointment or tincture) to reduce swelling and keep veins healthy. Try hawthorn, *Ginkgo biloba,* or bilberry to build up blood vessels and increase circulation. Eat garlic, cayenne, or ginger to keep legs soft and smooth.

HOMEOPATHY

To relieve swollen and painful varicose veins Belladonna 6C (Nightshade) or Carbo Vegetablis 6C (Vegetable Charcoal) seem to be the remedies that yield the best results. Hamamelis Virginica 6C (witch hazel) causes relaxation in the veins and relieves swelling.

MIND-BODY

To prevent varicose veins from spreading any further, bathe your feet in hot and cold baths: Place in warm water for one to two minutes, then put them in cold water for thirty seconds and keep switching for fifteen minutes. Try yoga, or take an aerobics class, power walk, or swim at least thirty minutes a day, three times a week to keep veins healthy and strong and improve circulation. Also, keep your weight down and wear loose clothing to eliminate constriction.

NUTRITION AND DIET

Try to avoid salt, sugar, and fat, bulk up on fiber (to prevent straining when you go to the bathroom). And don't smoke! You should drink at least eight glasses of water a day and eat more fruits, vegetables, and grains. Adding the bioflavonoid rutin as a supplement or in foods such as buckwheat, oranges, blueberries, blackberries, or cherries helps strengthen veins. Vitamin C and E supplements help keep blood vessels healthy.

REFLEXOLOGY

Reflexology can relieve you of pain if you focus on these points—sciatic nerve, digestive system, adrenal and parathyroid gland, heart, and liver.

Prevention

Try to keep pressure off veins in your pelvic area by sleeping on your left side if you're pregnant. Get plenty of exercise, and avoid fat, sugar, and salt.

Bath Basics

For a relaxing bath, the best (and safest) water temperature is a little warmer than body temperature. Add warm water as your bath begins to cool down, but keep your dip to less than half an hour: If you soak too long, you risk drying out your skin. Try one of the many bath milks, oils, and gels formulated to soften skin. After the bath, pat yourself almost dry with a big fluffy towel and use your favorite lotion or body oil to retain moisture in your skin.

If you're looking for added healing benefits from your bath, visit a naturopath or an aromatherapist for guidance. Consult an aromatherapy book for bath recipes or try one of the formulas below. Most of the herbs and aromatherapy oils are available at health food stores, herb shops, and bath boutiques.

RELAXING BATH

Add several drops of lavender and chamomile oils, or brew the dried herbs as a tea and add to bath water. Drink a cup of chamomile tea while soaking in this bath to promote a good night's sleep. After the bath, put a few drops of lavender on your pillow to invite sweet dreams.

FLU BATH

Add ½ cup of Epsom salts and several drops of eucalyptus oil to warm bath water; soak for fifteen minutes to thirty minutes. Drink a cup of peppermint tea during the bath to help clear the sinuses.

ENERGIZER BATH

Add several drops of lemon, grapefruit, wintergreen, peppermint, or rosemary oil to the water. Take a cool shower after the bath to stimulate circulation. Drink a cup of ginseng tea.

SCENTUAL BATH

Add sandalwood, ylang ylang, neroli, and/or rose to the water. Submerge and fantasize. Make sure someone is waiting for you when you come out of the bath!

Yeast Infection

Ladies, there are many folk remedies you may have heard from your mother or grandmother for treating yeast infections. We've included some that may actually help you with this problem. A yeast infection is an infection of the vagina or sometimes other body parts, usually caused by a fungus called *Candida albicans.* Candida is normally present in the vagina, mouth, intestines, and on the skin, but when the body's normally slightly acidic environment is too alkaline, the fungus can overgrow. Typical triggers include hormonal changes, antibiotics, douching, pregnancy, stress, diabetes, birth control pills, spermicides, and immune-compromising illnesses (AIDS, lupus). Vaginal symptoms include itching; odorless white discharge resembling cottage cheese; redness and swelling in vaginal area; soreness; and a burning sensation, especially during intercourse. A yeast infection in the mouth is called thrush; and it causes soreness, redness, and cottage cheese-like curds on the tongue. On the skin, a yeast infection appears as an inflamed rash that can infect the fingernails.

Statistics

Yeast infections affect over 30 million men and women every day.

Treatments

AROMATHERAPY

Tea tree oil and myrrh combat yeast infections of the skin. Add five drops to your bath. For itching and redness, add to your bath two drops essential oil of peppermint and four drops German chamomile, then bathe the affected area.

FOLK REMEDIES

Although unproven, the following are two home remedies that can relieve the discomfort of yeast infections. Douche with vinegar or yogurt solutions to restore natural pH and "good" bacteria. For vinegar douche, add 1 to 3 tablespoons white vinegar to 1 quart warm water; for yogurt douche, use live culture, plain *Lactobacillus acidophilus* yogurt and dilute with warm water. Douche for ten minutes.

HERBAL REMEDIES

A few suggestions for herbal treatments of yeast infection (of course, consult with a trained herbalist first): Diluted tea tree oil applied to the affected area helps relieve itchiness. For a vaginal yeast infection, coat the top half of a tampon with a lubricant (KY Jelly works well), then apply a few drops of tea tree oil on the tampon and insert in your vagina. Garlic is also an effective antifungal agent. Use it in your cooking or take in capsule form. Caprylic acid (extract of coconut) is another antifungal agent. For itching, bathe the vagina with a chickweed infusion. Pour 1 cup boiling water on 2 teaspoons herb, leave to infuse for five minutes, and allow to cool.

MIND-BODY

Learn how to manage stress: delegate and prioritize! Or try this technique: Close your eyes for five minutes and take an imaginary vacation to get away from it all. Use meditation and biofeedback for relaxation, too—it really works. Try alternating warm and cold sitz baths: sit in hot water for three minutes with a towel on the bottom of tub. Then sit in the cold bath for thirty seconds. Do this three times, ending with the cold bath.

NUTRITION AND DIET

Eat 1 cup of plain, live culture yogurt every day or take *Lactobacillus acidophilus* (½ teaspoon, three times a day). Cut down on sugar. Avoid raw, fresh fruits, alcohol, mushrooms, blue cheese, soy sauce (for one month), coffee, and tea. Eat lots of olive oil (to fight bacteria), fresh vegetables, whole-grain cereals, lean meat and fish. Drink mineral water, rooibos tea, and herbal teas.

Prevention

To keep yeast infections from coming back, wear all-cotton underwear, loose clothing made of natural fabric, and avoid wearing tight clothing and pantyhose. Avoid commercial douches, afterbath powders made of talc, cornstarch, bubble bath, colored toilet paper, and scented tampons. Wash before lovemaking; practice good oral hygiene; and always keep your genital area dry. You might want to consider barrier-type contraceptives (such as a condom or diaphragm) instead of birth control pills. Also, use pads instead of tampons to reduce the risk of the spread of infection.

Holistic Health Resource Guide

- *African Holistic Health* (Sea Island Information Group, $14.95) by Llaila O. Afrika
  The first reference book of its kind on African holistic healing, this is a complete herbal remedy guide discussing disease, diet, nutrition and other health concerns.
- *Aromatherapy* (Element Books, $9.95) by Christine Wildwood
  A look at how massaging with essential oils can lead to better health.
- *Aromatherapy Workbook* (Healing Arts Press, $12.95) by Marcel Lavabre
  A practical guide to the use of essential oils, featuring more than seventy oils, with detailed discussions of their specific actions and healing properties.
- *The Book of Massage* (Simon & Schuster, $14) by Lucinda Lidell and Sara Thomas
  A step-by-step guide to hands-on healing techniques, including massage reflexology.
- *Chinese Medicine* (Element Books, $9.95) by Tom Williams, Ph.D.
  A discussion of the uses of acupuncture, herbal remedies, nutrition, Chi gong, and meditation.
- *The Encyclopedia of Essential Oils* (Element Books, $14.95) by Julia Lawless
  A complete guide to the use of aromatics in aromatherapy, herbal health, and well-being.

Bibliography

The African Background to Medical Science by Charles S. Finch, Ph.D., Karnak House, 1990.

African Religions: Symbol, Ritual, and Community by B.C. Ray, Prentice-Hall, 1976.

The Alternative Advisor, Time-Life Books, 1997.

The Alternative Health & Medicine Encyclopedia by James E. Marti, Visible Ink, 1988.

Alternative Medicine: The Definitive Guide by Leon Chaitow, N.D., D.O., Future Medicine, 1995.

Aromathérapie by Jean Valet, 1965.

Aromatherapy: Massage with Essential Oils, by Christine Wildwood, Element Books, 1998.

Aromatherapy Workbook by Marcel Lavabre, Healing Arts Press, 1990.

Art of Reflexology: A Step-by-Step Guide by Inge Dougans with Suzzane Ellis, Element Books, 1992.

Biochemical Individuality by Roger Williams Ph.D., University of Texas Press, 1980.

Body and Soul: The Black Women's Guide to Physical Health and Emotional Well-being, edited by Linda Villarosa, Harper Perennial, 1994.

The Book of Massage by Lucinda Lidell and Sara Thomas, Simon & Schuster, 1984.

Chinese Medicine by Tom Williams, Ph.D., Element Books.

Colon Health: Key to a Vibrant Life by Norman Walker, Norwalk Press, 1995.

Everybody's Guide to Homeopathic Medicine: Safe and Effective Remedies for You and Your Family by Stephen Cummings, M.D., and Dana Ullman, M.P.H., Putnam Publishing Group, 1997.

The Family Guide to Homeopathy: Symptoms and Natural Solutions by Dr. Andrew Lockie, Fireside, 1993.

Heal Thyself for Health and Longevity by Queen Afua, A&B Books, 1998.

The Healing Foods: The Ultimate Authority on the Curative Power of Nutrition by Patricia Hausman and Judith Benn Hurley, Dell Publishing, 1991.

The Healing Herbs by Michael Castleman, Bantam Books, 1995.

Healing and the Mind by David Smith, M.D., Doubleday, 1993.

The Healing Source by Wilson Bactuu, Wilson-Derek.

Healing with Homeopathy: The Complete Guide by Wayne B. Jonas and Jennifer Jacobs, Warner Books, 1996.

Healing With Homeopathy: The Natural Way to Promote Recovery and Restore Health by Wayne Jonas, JMD, and Jennifer Jacobs, M.D., M.P.H., Warner Books, 1996.

Healing Within: The Complete Colon Health Guide by Stanley Weinberger, Healing Within Products, 1988.

Healing Words: The Power of Prayer and the Practice of Medicine by Larry Dossey, M.D., HarperCollins, 1994.

Herbal and Magical Medicine by Holly F. Mathews, Ph.D., Duke University Press, 1993.

Herbal Medicine: The Use of Herbs for Health and Healing by Vicki Pittman, Element Books, 1995.

Homeopathic Medicine at Home: Natural Remedies for Everyday Ailments and Minor Injuries by Maesimund B. Panos, M.D., and Jane Heimlich, Jeremy Tarcher, Inc., 1980.

Homeopathy: Medicine for the 21st Century by Robert Ullman, N.D. and Judith Reichenberg Ullman, N.D.

How to Get Well by Pavlo Airola, Health Plus, 1974.

The Illustrated Encyclopedia of Essential Oils: The Complete Guide to the Use of Oils in Aromatherapy and Herbalism by Julia Lawless, Element Books, 1995.

In the Company of My Sisters: Black Women and Self-Esteem by Julia Boyd, Dutton, 1993.

Medicinal Resources of the Tropical Forest, Columbia University Press, 1996.

Nature's Pharmacy: A History of Plants and Healing by Christine Stockwell, Century, 1988.

Nerys Purchon's Handbook of Natural Healing by Nerys Pruchon, A Sue Hines Book, Allen & Unwin pty Ltd, 1998.

New Choices in Natural Healing, Rodale Press, 1995.

Prescription for Nutritional Healing: A Practical A-Z Reference to Drug-Free Remedies Using Vitmains, Herbs and Food Supplements by James Balch, M.D., and Phyllis A. Balch, C.N.C., Avery Publishing Group.

A Path to Healing: A Guide to Wellness for Body, Mind and Soul by Andrea Sullivan, N.D., Doubleday, 1998.

Roll, Jordan, Roll by Eugene D. Genovese, Ph.D., Pantheon Books, 1974.

The Self-Healing Workbook: Your Personal Plan for Stress-Free Living by C. Norman Shealry, M.D., Ph.D., Element Books, 1993.

Spontaneous Healing by Andrew Weil, M.D., Alfred Knopf, 1995.

Stories the Feet Can Tell Thru Reflexology by Eunice Ingham, Ingham Publishing, 1984.

Walkin' Over Medicine by Loudell Snow, Ph.D., Westview Press, 1993.

West African Traditional Religion by Kofi Asare Opoku, FEP International, 1978.

The Women's Guide to Homeopathy by Andrew Lockie, M.D., and Nicola Geddes, M.D., St. Martin's Press, 1994.

Yellow Emperor's Classic of Internal Medicine by Ilza Veith, University of California Press, 1966.

Index